| Chapter | Chapter Title | Video Contributor | Video Title |
|---|---|---|---|
| 1 | Clinical Examination and Imaging of the Hip | Hal Martin, MD | Physical Exam of the Adult and Adolescent Hip |
| 2 | Chondral Lesions | Corey A. Wolf, MD and Christopher Larson, MD | Hip Arthroscopy: Management of Chondral Lesions |
| 3 | Labral Pathology | Carlos A. Gaunche, MD, Ivan H. Wong, MD and James P. Sieradzki, MD | Arthroscopic Debridement of Pincer Impingement and Labral Repair |
| 4 | Femoroacetabular Impingement - Cam | J. W. Thomas Byrd, MD | Arthroscopic Femoroplasty: Correction of Cam Lesion |
| 9 | External Snapping Hip Syndrome | Victor M. Ilizaliturri, Jr., MD | Endoscopic Release of the Endotibial Band |
| 10 | Adbuctor Tears | William J. Robertson, MD, Anil Ranawat, MD and Bryan T. Kelly, MD | Arthroscopic Treatment of Peritrochanteric Space Disorders of the Hip |

AANA Advanced Arthroscopy

# The Hip

*Series Editor*

## Richard K. N. Ryu, MD

President (2009-2010)
Arthroscopy Association of North America
Private Practice
Santa Barbara, California

---

## Other Volumes in the AANA Advanced Arthroscopy Series

### The Foot and Ankle

### The Elbow and Wrist

### The Knee

### The Shoulder

## AANA Advanced Arthroscopy

# The Hip

**J.W. Thomas Byrd, MD**
Nashville Sports Medicine Foundation
Nashville, Tennessee

**Carlos A. Guanche, MD**
Southern California Orthopaedic Institute
Van Nuys, California

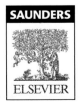

SAUNDERS

ELSEVIER

**SAUNDERS**
ELSEVIER

1600 John F. Kennedy Blvd.
Ste 1800
Philadelphia, PA 19103-2899

AANA Advanced Arthroscopy: The Hip

ISBN: 978-1-4377-0911-7

---

**Notice**

Knowledge and best practice in this field are constantly changing. As new research and experience broaden our knowledge, changes in practice, treatment and drug therapy may become necessary or appropriate. Readers are advised to check the most current information provided (i) on procedures featured or (ii) by the manufacturer of each product to be administered to verify the recommended dose or formula, the method and duration of administration, and contraindications. It is the responsibility of the practitioner, relying on their own experience and knowledge of the patient, to make diagnoses, to determine dosages and the best treatment for each individual patient, and to take all appropriate safety precautions. To the fullest extent of the law, neither the Publisher nor the Authors assumes any liability for any injury and/or damage to persons or property arising out of or related to any use of the material contained in this book.

The Publisher

---

**Library of Congress Cataloging-in-Publication Data**
AANA advanced arthroscopy. the hip / [edited by] J.W. Thomas Byrd, Carlos A. Guanche. -- 1st ed.
        p. ; cm.
   Other title: Advanced arthroscopy
   Other title: Hip
   Includes bibliographical references.
   ISBN 978-1-4377-0911-7
   1. Hip joint Endoscopic surgery.   I. Byrd, J. W. Thomas (John Wilson Thomas), 1957-
II. Guanche, Carlos A.   III. Arthroscopy Association of North America.   IV. Title: Advanced arthroscopy.   V. Title: Hip.
   [DNLM: 1.   Hip Joint--surgery.   2.   Arthroscopy--methods.   WE 860 A112 2010]
   RD549.A16 2010
   617.5'810597--dc22                                                  2010011088

*Publishing Director:* Kim Murphy
*Developmental Editor:* Ann Ruzycka Anderson
*Publishing Services Manager:* Frank Polizzano
*Senior Project Manager:* Peter Faber
*Design Direction:* Ellen Zanolle

Printed in China

Last digit is the print number:  9  8  7  6  5  4  3  2

## DEDICATION

*To my loving wife, Donna, and wonderful daughters, Allison and Ellen, whose patience and understanding have allowed me to tackle projects like this. Also, to Kay and Sharon, and the entire Nashville Sports Medicine staff, whose dedication has been integral to everything we have done together in patient care, education and research. Thanks to them all.*

**J. W. Thomas Byrd, MD**

---

*To my wonderful wife, Anna, and my children, Carlos and Isabella. Thanks for your support and understanding with all of these projects.*

**Carlos Guanche, MD**

# Contributors

**Asheesh, Bedi, MD**
Assistant Professor, Sports Medicine and Shoulder Surgery, Medsports, University of Michigan, Ann Arbor, Michigan
*Abductor Tears; Clinical Examination and Imaging of the Hip*

**J. W. Thomas Byrd, MD**
Nashville Sports Medicine Foundation, Nashville, Tennessee
*Cam-Type Femoroacetabular Impingement*

**Mrs. Laurence Chabanas**
A² Surgical, Grenoble, France
*Computer-Assisted Surgery for Femoroacetabular Impingement*

**Carlos A. Guanche, MD**
Southern California Orthopedic Institute
Van Nuys, California
*Labral Pathology; Hip Instability*

**Victor M. Ilizaliturri, Jr., MD**
Professor, Knee and Hip Surgery, Universidad Nacional Autónoma de México; Instituto Nacional de Rehabilitación; Chief, Hip and Knee Adult Joint Reconstruction, National Rehabilitation Institute of México, Mexico City, Mexico
*External Snapping Hip Syndrome*

**Sunil Jani, MD**
Resident, Department of Orthopedic Surgery, University of Pennsylvania, Philadelphia, Pennsylvania
*Internal Snapping Hip Syndrome*

**Bryan T. Kelly, MD**
Attending Orthopedic Surgeon, Hospital for Special Surgery, New York, New York
*Abductor Tears; Compute-Assisted Surgery for Femoroacetabular Impingement*

**Christopher M. Larson, MD**
Education Director, Minnesota Orthopedic Sports Medicine Institute, Minneapolis, Minnesota
*Chondral Lesions*

**Séphane Lavallée**
A² Surgical, Grenoble, France
*Computer-Assisted Surgery for Femoroacetabular Impingement*

**Hal David Martin, DO**
The Hip Clinic, Sports Science and Orthopedics, Oklahoma City, Oklahoma
*Clinical Examination and Imaging of the Hip*

**Marc J. Philippon, MD**
Clinical Professor, University of Pittsburgh Medical Center for Sports Medicine; Medical Consultant, National Hockey League Players Association, Orthopedic Surgeon, Steadman Clinic, Vail, Colorado
*Femoroacetabular Impingement: Pince*

**Marc R. Safran, MD**
Professor, Orthopedic Surgery, Stanford University; Associate Director, Sports Medicine, Stanford University Hospital and Clinics, Redwood City, California
*Internal Snapping Hip Syndrome*

**Thomas G. Sampson, MD**
Medical Director Total Joint Center, Saint Francis Memorial Hospital; Director, Hip Arthroscopy, Post Street Surgery Center, San Francisco, California
*Miscellaneous Problems: Synovitis, Degenerative Joint Disease, and Tumors*

**Bruno G. Schröder e Souza, MD**
Visiting Scholar in Hip Arthroscopy and Biomechanics,
Steadman Hawkins Research Foundation, Vail, Colorado
*Femoroacetabular Impingement: Pincer*

**Jérome Tonetti, MD**
Professor, Department of Orthopedics, Marchallon Hospital,
Université Joseph Fourier, Grenoble, France
*Computer-Assisted Surgery for Femoroacetabular Impingement*

**Ivan Ho Wong, MD, PhD**
Associate Professor, Department of Orthopedic Surgery,
Samsung Medical Center, Sungkyunkwan University School
of Medicine, Seoul, Korea
*Labral Pathology*

**Corey A. Wulf, MD**
Clinical Professor, Sanford School, University of South Dakota,
Vermillion, South Dakota
*Chondral Lesions*

# Preface

The Arthroscopy Association of North America (AANA) is a robust and growing organization whose mission, simply stated, is to provide leadership and expertise in arthroscopic and minimally invasive surgery worldwide.

Towards that end, this five-volume series represents the very best that AANA has to offer the clinician in need of a timely, authoritative, and comprehensive arthroscopic textbook. These textbooks covering the shoulder, elbow and wrist, hip, knee, and foot and ankle were conceived and rapidly consummated over a 15-month timeline. The need for an up-to-date and cogent text as well as a step-by-step video supplement was the driving force behind the rapid developmental chronology. The topics and surgical techniques represent the cutting edge in arthroscopic philosophy and technique, and the individual chapters follow a reliable and helpful format in which the pathoanatomy is detailed and the key elements of the physical examination are emphasized in conjunction with preferred diagnostic imaging. Indications and contraindications are followed by a thorough discussion of the treatment algorithm, both nonoperative and surgical, with an emphasis on arthroscopic techniques. Additionally, a Pearls and Pitfalls section provides for a distilled summary of the most important features in each chapter. A brief annotated bibliography is provided in addition to a comprehensive reference list so that those who want to study the most compelling literature can do so with ease. The supporting DVD meticulously demonstrates the surgical techniques, and will undoubtedly serve as a critical resource in preparing for any arthroscopic intervention.

I am most grateful for the outstanding effort provided by the volume editors: Rick Angelo and Jim Esch (shoulder), Buddy Savoie and Larry Field (elbow and wrist), Thomas Byrd and Carlos Guanche (hip), Rob Hunter and Nick Sgaglione (knee), and Ned Amendola and Jim Stone (foot and ankle). Their collective intellect, skill, and dedicaton to AANA made this series possible. Furthermore, I sincerely thank all the chapter contributors whose expertise and wisdom can be found in every page. Elsevier, and in particular Kim Murphy, Ann Ruzycka Anderson, and Kitty Lasinski, was a delight to work with, and deserves our gratitude for a job well done. I would be remiss if I did not acknowledge that the proceeds of this five-volume series will go directly to the AANA Education Foundation, from which ambitious and state-of-the-art arthroscopic educational initiatives will be funded.

RICHARD K.N. RYU, MD
Series Editor

# Contents

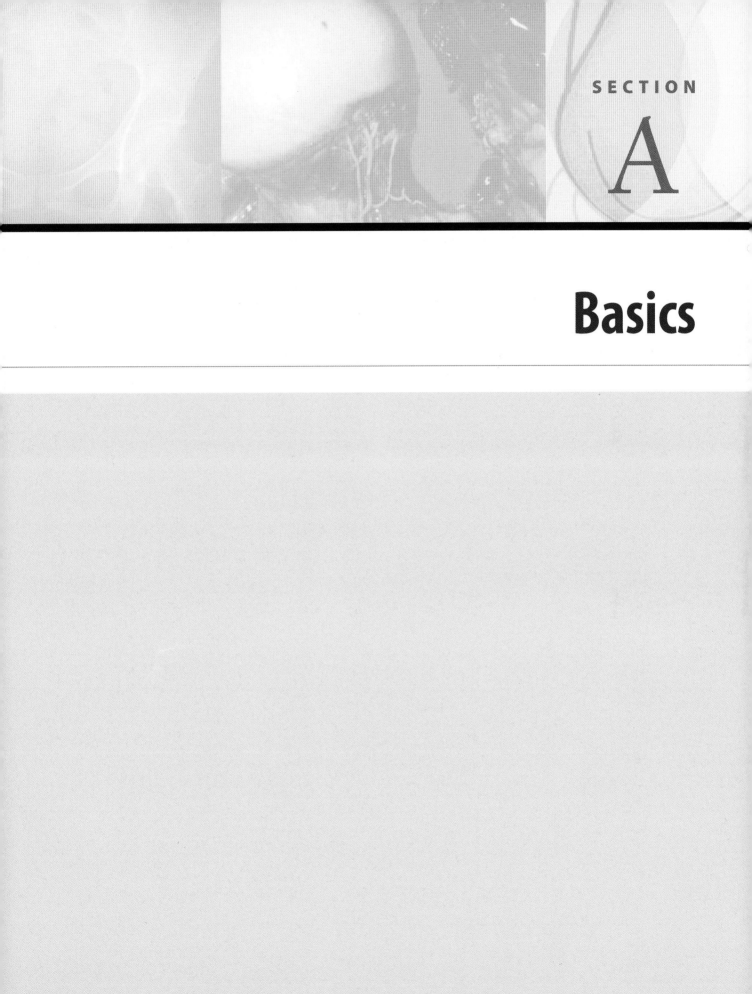

# Basics

# Clinical Examination and Imaging of the Hip

Hal David Martin

The clinical examination of the hip is a comprehensive assessment of osseous, ligamentous, and musculotendinous tissues. To appreciate this achievement of symphonic function, it is important to understand the balance and interrelationships of each system with the other in a static and dynamic fashion. Imaging of the hip is a powerful tool for the visualization and quantification of the structures within and about the hip joint. Imaging techniques continue to evolve as our understanding of pathologic hip conditions advances. Optimally, the hip will be recognized early as the source of the complaint, which is dependent on a consistent method of interpreting the history, clinical examination, and imaging of the hip. The goal of this chapter will be to describe in detail how to perform the clinical examination of the hip and explain why these tests are important, raise awareness for commonly found but uncommonly recognized conditions, and describe the current methodologies for accurate diagnostic imaging.

## HISTORY AND PHYSICAL EXAMINATION

### History

Prior to the physical examination of the hip, the patient history is recorded. An account of the present condition, including the date of onset, the presence or absence of trauma, mechanisms of injury, pain location, and factors that increase or decrease the pain, is obtained. Treatments to date must be clearly defined, such as rest, physical therapy, ice, heat, nonsteroidal anti-inflammatory drugs (NSAIDs), surgery, injections, orthotics, and/or the use of support aids. The patient's functional status is assessed and current limitations are detailed, which may involve getting in or out of a bathtub or car,

activities of daily living, jogging, walking, and/or climbing stairs. Related symptoms of the back and neurologic, abdomen, and lower extremity complaints must also be identified. The presence of associated complaints, such as abdominal or back pain, numbness, weakness, sitting pain, length of time sitting, and coughing or sneezing exacerbation, help rule out thoracolumbar problems. Previous consultations, surgical interventions, and past injuries must also be addressed.

The location of the presenting pain and presence or absence of popping will aid in the determination of intra-articular versus extra-articular causes. Participation in sports and other activities are documented, which can help determine the type of injury. Rotation sports, such as golf, tennis, ballet, and martial arts, have been commonly associated with injuries to the intra-articular structures. Finally, treatment goals and expectations are reviewed with the patient. Treatment may vary, based on the patient's expectations and postoperative goals. See Figure 1-1 for an illustration of a form for a complete review of the history.

A modified Harris hip or Merle d'Aubigné (MDA) score is a general guide to establish the gross levels of function. The modified Harris hip score (HHS) is the most documented and standardized functional score to date, which is a quantitative score based on pain and function. However, the high-performing athletic population may be best evaluated by the athletic hip score.[1] Other hip scores have been outlined with quantifications for more specific patient populations, such as the nonarthritic hip score (NAHS), hip disability and osteoarthritis outcome score (HOOS), musculoskeletal function assessment (MFA), short form 36 (SF-36), and the Western Ontario and McMaster University (WOMAC) osteoarthritis index.[2] Currently, the

NAME: _____

DATE: _____

AGE: _____

EMPLOYMENT: _____

REFERRED BY: _____

CHIEF COMPLAINT:    L HIP    R HIP    OTHER: _____

**HISTORY OF PRESENT ILLNESS:**

- Date of onset _____
- Pain location _____
- Traumatic/nontraumatic
- Have you ever been diagnosed with AVN? If yes, do you have a family history of heart disease, stroke, or clotting disorders? _____
  Alcohol use _____    Tobacco use _____    Steroid use _____
  Labs: Homocysteine ____    Factor V Leiden _____    Lipid profile _____    Thyroid profile _____
- Pain a.m./p.m.          popping/locking

- Mechanism of injury_____
- Pain increased with _____
- Pain decreased with _____

**TREATMENT TO DATE**

Rest    Ice    Heat    NSAIDS _____

PT_____

Surgery_____

Chiropractic tx _____

Injections _____

Support (cane, crutch) _____

Orthotics_____

**TEST AND EVALUATIONS:**

MRI    MRI Arthrogram    X-rays    Lab    Biometrics    Consults _____

**PAST INJURIES:** _____

**LIMITATIONS:**

- Sitting                    Length of Time able to sit _____
- Getting in or out of car
- Getting in or out of tub        • Stairs
- Sports                    • Work
- Jogging                   • ADL's
- Walking                   • Household activities

**FUNCTION:**

HHS _____    VAS:    Pain at rest (0–10) _____
                            Pain with activity_____

**ASSOCIATED**

- Back        L        R            • Weakness
- Night pain awakening
- 
- Numbness

**SPORTS AND ACTIVITIES:** _____

**GOAL IN TREATMENT:** _____

**REVIEW OF SYSTEMS:**

**FIGURE 1-1** Complete review of patient history.

MAHORN (Multicenter Arthroscopy of the Hip Outcomes Research Network) Group is in the final stages of testing the hip outcomes score (HOS), which will provide an internationally accepted score and be useful for the athletic population.[3]

## Physical Examination

The hip assumes an essential role in most activities. The hip is not only responsible for distributing weight between the appendicular and axial skeleton, but is also the joint from which motion is initiated and executed. It is known that the forces through the hip joint can reach three to five times the body's weight during running and jumping.[4] Hip pain often stems from some type of sports-related injury.[1] Of athletic injuries in children, 10% to 24% are hip-related, whereas 5%

to 6% of adult sports injuries originate in the hip and pelvis.[5] Athletes participating in rugby and martial arts have also been reported to have an increased incidence of degenerative hip disease.[6] Currently, 60% of intra-articular disorders are initially misdiagnosed.[7] An organized physical examination will help in the diagnosis of hip problems.

A consistent hip examination is performed quickly and efficiently to screen the hip, back, and abdominal, neurovascular, and neurologic systems and to find the comorbidities that coexist with complex hip pathology. Each examination or physical evaluation has a specific method of being performed, although interobserver consistency and practice is one of the most important aspects of the evaluation.[8]

The technique of physical examination is dependent on the examiner's experience and efficiency. The most efficient order of examination begins with standing tests followed by seated, supine, and lateral tests, ending with prone tests.[9,10] The physical examination will be fine-tuned and directed through the review of the history of present illness. As with other extremity examinations, access for exposure and patient comfort with loose-fitting clothes about the waist are helpful. An assistant to record the examination on a standardized written form aids in accurate documentation and thoroughness, especially when first starting a comprehensive hip evaluation.

Recently, the MAHORN Group has identified common trends among hip specialists in the physical examination of the hip. In the standing position, common tests included gait analysis, single-leg stance phase test, and laxity. In the supine position, common tests included the following: range of motion (ROM) of hip flexion; internal and external hip ROM; flexion, adduction, internal rotation (FADDIR); dynamic internal rotatory impingement (DIRI); dynamic external rotatory impingement (DEXRIT); palpation, flexion, abduction, external rotation (FABER); straight leg raise against resistance; muscular strength; passive supine rotation; and posterior rim impingement. Common lateral position tests included palpation, passive adduction tests, and abductor strength. In the prone position, the femoral anteversion test was commonly performed. The physical examination that follows includes these points.

### Standing Examination

As the patient stands (Table 1-1), a general point of pain is noted with one finger, and can usually help direct the examination. The groin region directs a suspicion of intra-articular problem and lateral-based pain is primarily associated with intra- or extra-articular aspects. A characteristic sign of patients with intra-articular hip pain is the C sign.[8] The patient will hold his or her hand in the shape of a C and place it above the greater trochanter, with the thumb positioned posterior to the trochanter and fingers extending into the groin. This finding can be misinterpreted as lateral soft tissue pathology, such as trochan-

teric bursitis or the iliotibial band; however, the patient is often describing deep interior hip pain.[8] Posterior-superior pain requires a thorough evaluation in differentiating hip and back pain. The shoulder height and iliac crest heights are noted to evaluate leg length discrepancies (Fig. 1-2). Incremental wooden blocks placed under the short side heel help in orthotic considerations. General body habitus is assessed and issues of ligamentous laxity are determined by the middle finger test or hyperextension of the elbows or knees. Structural versus nonstructural scoliosis is differentiated by forward bending and the degree of lumbar flexion is recorded. Side-bending ROM is also useful.

Gait abnormalities often help detect hip pathology.[11,12] Joint stability, preservation of the labrum and articular cartilage, and proper functioning of the hip joint involve three biomechanical planes of the femur and acetabulum. These relationships are important for the transfer of dynamic and static load to the ligamentous and osseous structures.

The patient is taken into the hallway to observe a full gait of six to eight stride lengths. Key points of gait evaluation include foot rotation (internal-external progression angle), pelvic rotation in the x and y axes, stance phase, and stride length. Gait viewed from the foot progression angle will detect osseous or static rotatory malalignment, such as that which exists with increased or decreased femoral anteversion versus capsular or musculotendinous issues. The knee and thigh are observed simultaneously to assess any rotatory parameters. The knee may want to be held in internal or external rotation to allow proper patellofemoral joint alignment, but may produce a secondary abnormal hip rotation. This abnormal motion is usually present in cases of severe increased femoral anteversion, precipitating a battle between the hip and knee for a comfortable position, which will affect the gait. In cases of a painful gait, note the anatomic location of pain and at what point within the gait phase pain is manifest.

Noting iliac crest rotation and terminal hip extension assesses pelvic rotation. On average, a normal gait requires 6 to 8 degrees of hip rotation and 7 degrees of pelvic rotation, for a

---

**TABLE 1-1** Standing Examination Assessment

| Examination | Assessment and Association |
|---|---|
| Abductor deficient gait | Abductor strength, proprioception mechanism |
| Antalgic | Trauma, fracture, synovial inflammation |
| Pelvic rotational wink | Intra-articular pathology, hip flexion contracture, increased femoral anteversion, anterior capsual laxity |
| Foot progression angle with excessive external rotation | Femoral retroversion, increased acetabular anteversion, torsional abnormalities, effusion, ligamentous injury |
| Foot progression angle with excessive internal rotation | Increased femoral anteversion or acetabular retroversion, torsional abnormalities |
| Short leg limp | Iliotibial band pathology, true-false leg length discrepancy |
| Single-leg stance phase test | Abductor strength, proprioception mechanism |
| Spinal alignment | Shoulder–iliac crest heights, lordosis, scoliosis, leg length |
| Laxity | Ligamentous laxity in other joints: thumb, elbows, shoulders, or knee |

*See video for performing seated examination tests.*

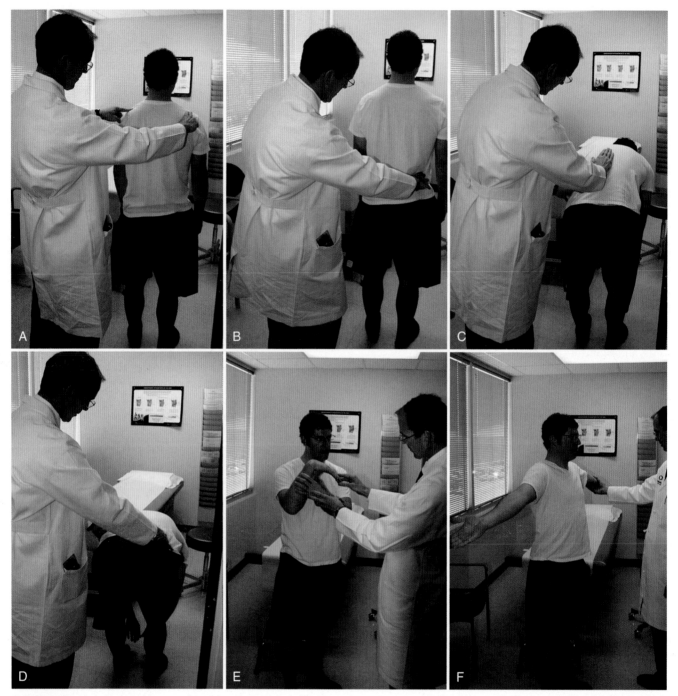

**FIGURE 1-2** Body habitus and laxity evaluation. **A, B,** Shoulder and iliac crest heights are examined with the patient with dynamic loading of the hip joint in the standing position. **C,** As the patient bends forward at the trunk, spinal alignment is palpated. **D,** The degree of truncal flexion is noted in full flexion. **E,** Laxity of the thumb. **F,** Recurvatum of the elbow.

total rotation of 15 degrees.[12] The pelvic wink is demonstrated by an excessive rotation in the axial plane toward the affected hip, thus producing extension and rotation through the lumbar spine, to obtain terminal hip extension. This winking gait can be associated with intra-articular hip pathology, laxity, or hip flexion contractures, especially when combined with increased lumbar lordosis or a forward-stooping posture. Gait changes can affect spinal mechanics and function. Excessive femoral anteversion, or retroversion, can affect a wink on terminal hip

extension because the patient will try to create greater anterior coverage with a rotated pelvis. Injury to the anterior capsule can also contribute to a winking gait.

During the stance phase, body weight must be supported by a single leg, with the gluteus maximus, medius, and minimus providing most of the force.[12] Maximum ground reactive force occurs on heel strike at 30 degrees of hip flexion. A shortened stance phase can be indicative of neuromuscular abnormalities, trauma, or leg length discrepancies.

The abductor deficient gait (Trendelenburg gait or abductor lurch) is an unbalanced stance phase attributed to abductor weakness or proprioception disruption. This pattern may present in two ways—with a shift of the pelvis away from the body (a dropping out of the hip on the affected side), or with a shift of the weight over the adducted leg (a shift of the upper body over the top of the affected hip). The antalgic gait is characterized by a shortened stance phase on the painful side, limiting the duration of weight-bearing (a self-protecting limp caused by pain). A short leg gait is noted by drop of the shoulder in the direction of the short leg.

In addition to body habitus and gait evaluation, the single-leg stance phase test (Trendelenburg test) is performed during the standing evaluation of the hip. The single-leg stance phase test is performed on both legs, with the nonaffected leg examined first, to establish a baseline (Fig. 1-3). During this test, the examiner stands behind the exposed patient (to the degree that the bony landmarks are easily observed). The patient stands with the feet shoulder width apart and then brings one leg forward by flexing the leg to 45 degrees at the hip and 45 degrees at the knee, thereby simulating the single-leg stance phase with the load on the examined hip. This position is held for 6 seconds. As the patient lifts and holds one foot off the ground, the contralateral hip abductor musculature and neural loop of proprioception are being tested. The pelvis will tilt toward or away from the unsupported side if the musculature is weak or if the neural loop of proprioception is disrupted. Normal dynamic midstance translocation is 2 cm during a normal gait pattern[12]; a shift in either direction of more than 2 cm constitutes a positive shift. This test is also performed in a dynamic fashion by some examiners.

### Seated Examination

The seated hip examination (Table 1-2) consists of a thorough neurologic and vascular examination. The need to check the basics is obvious, even in apparently healthy individuals. The posterior tibial pulse is checked first, any swelling of the extremity is noted, and inspection of the skin is performed at this

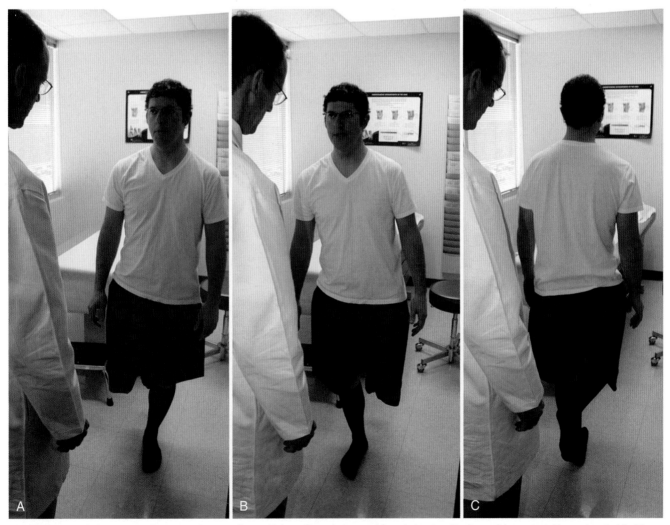

**FIGURE 1-3** Single-leg stance phase test. This is performed bilaterally and observed from behind and in front of the patient. The patient holds this position for 6 seconds. A pelvic shift of greater than 2 cm is a positive result, indicating abductor weakness or proprioception disruption. **A,** Left leg front view. **B,** Right leg, front view. **C,** Left leg, rear view.

time. A straight leg raise test is then performed by passively extending the knee into full extension. The straight leg raise test is helpful for detecting radicular neurologic symptoms.

The loss of internal rotation is one of the first signs of an intra-articular disorder; therefore, one of the most important

**TABLE 1-2**   Seated Examination Assessment

| Examination | Assessment and Association |
|---|---|
| Neurologic | Sensory nerves originating from the L2-S1 levels, deep tendon reflex of patella (L2-L4 spinal nerves and femoral nerve) and Achilles (L5-S1 sacral nerves) |
| Straight leg raise | Radicular neurologic symptoms |
| Vascular | Pulses of the dorsalis pedis and posterior tibial artery |
| Lymphatics | Skin inspection for swelling, scarring, or side to side asymmetry |
| Internal rotation | Normal between 20 and 35 degrees |
| External rotation | Normal between 30 and 45 degrees |

*See video for performing seated examination tests.*

assessments is internal and external rotation in the seated position. The seated position ensures that the ischium is square to the table, thus providing sufficient stability at 90 degrees of hip flexion and a reproducible platform for accurate rotational measurement. Passive internal and external rotation testing are performed gently and compared from side to side. Seated rotation range of motion is also compared and contrasted with the extended position of the hip (Fig. 1-4).

Musculotendinous, ligamentous, and osseous control of internal and external rotation are complex, so any differences in seated versus extended positions may raise the question of ligamentous versus osseous abnormality. Sufficient internal rotation is important for proper hip function—there should be at least 10 degrees of internal rotation at the midstance phase of normal gait,[12] but less than 20 degrees is abnormal (see Table 1-3 for normal ROM). Pathology related to femoro-acetabular impingement or to rotational constraint from increased or decreased femoral or acetabular anteversion can result in significant side-to-side differences. An increased internal rotation combined with a decreased external rotation may indicate excessive femoral anteversion and distinguished from hip capsular pathology by radiographic and biometric assessment.

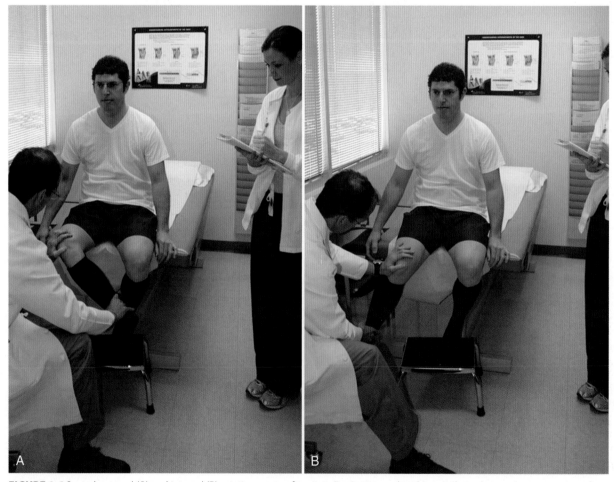

**FIGURE 1-4** Seated external (**A**) and internal (**B**) rotation range of motion. Passive internal and external rotation testing are compared from side to side. In the seated position, the ischium is square to the table, thus providing sufficient stability at 90 degrees of hip flexion. Internal and external rotation in the seated position offer a reproducible platform for the accurate rotational measurement.

**TABLE 1-3** Normal Internal and External Rotation Range of Motion

| Range of Motion Assessment | Normal (degrees) | Abnormal (degrees) |
|---|---|---|
| Seated internal rotation | 20-35 | <20 |
| Seated external rotation | 30-45 | <30 |
| Extended internal rotation | 20-35 | <20 |
| Extended external rotation | 30-45 | <30 |
| Supine hip flexion | 100-110 | <100 |
| Adduction | 20-30 | <20 |
| Abduction | 45 | <45 |

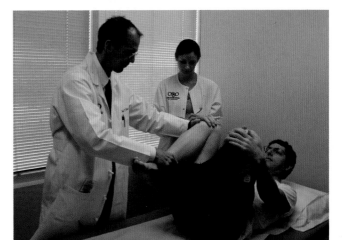

**FIGURE 1-5** Supine examination, starting position. Zero set point of the pelvis is achieved by having the patient hold the contralateral leg in full flexion, thus establishing neutral pelvic inclination.

## Supine Examination

A battery of tests with the patient in the supine position (Table 1-4) helps distinguish internal from extra-articular sources of hip symptoms further. The supine examination begins with the assessment of leg lengths. Next, passive hip flexion range of motion is assessed (Table 1-3). Both knees are brought up to the chest and the degree of flexion is recorded (Fig. 1-5). It is important to note the pelvic position because the hip may stop early in flexion, with the end range of motion being predominantly pelvic rotation. From this position, the hip flexion contracture test (Thomas test) is performed by having the patient extend and relax one leg down toward the table (Fig. 1-6). Any lack of terminal extension, noted by the inability of the thigh to reach the table, demonstrates a hip flexion contracture. Both sides are examined for comparison. An important aspect of this test is to obtain the zero set point for the lumbar spine. Patients with hyperlaxity or connective tissue disorders could have a false-negative result. In these patients, the zero set point can be established with an abdominal contraction. The hip flexion contracture test could also be falsely negative if there is lumbar spine hyperlordosis.

**TABLE 1-4** Summary of Supine Examinations and Assessment

| Examination | Assessment and Association |
|---|---|
| Range of motion | Flexion, abduction, adduction |
| FADDIR | Anterior femoroacetabular impingement, torn labrum |
| Hip flexion contracture test (Thomas test) | Hip flexor contracture (psoas), femoral neuropathy, intra-articular pathology, abdominal cause |
| FABER (Flexion, Abduction, External Rotation) | Distinguish between back and hip pathology, specifically sacroiliac joint pathology |
| Dynamic internal rotatory impingement test (similar to McCarthy test) | Anterior femoroacetabular impingement, torn labrum |
| Dynamic external rotatory impingement test (similar to McCarthy test) | Superior femoroacetabular impingement, torn labrum |
| Posterior rim impingement test | Posterior femoroacetabular impingement, torn labrum |
| Passive supine rotation test (log roll) | Trauma, effusion, synovitis |
| Heel strike | Trauma, femoral fracture |
| Straight leg raise against resistance (Stinchfield) | Intraarticular pathology along with psoas tendonitis or bursitis. Hip flexor strength |
| Palpation | |
|     Abdomen | Fascial hernia, associated gastrointestinal or genitourinary pathology |
|     Pubic symphysis | Osteitis pubis, calcification, fracture, trauma |
|     Adductor tubercle | Adductor tendinitis |

*See video for performing supine examination tests.*

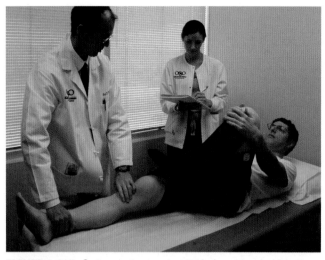

**FIGURE 1-6** Hip flexion contracture test. With the patient holding the contralateral leg in full flexion (zero set point for the lumbar spine), the examined hip is passively extended toward the table. Both hips are examined for side to side comparison. If the thigh cannot reach the table (lack of terminal hip extension), this demonstrates a hip flexion contracture.

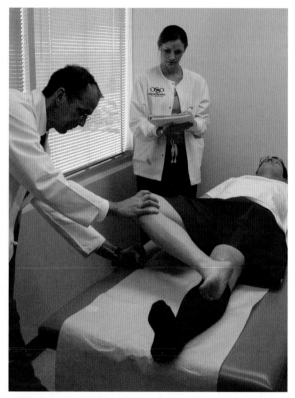

**FIGURE 1-7** Flexion, abduction, external rotation test (FABER) test. The examiner brings the leg into 90 degrees of flexion and externally rotates and abducts it so that the ipsilateral ankle rests distal to the knee of the contralateral leg. The passive abduction ROM can be measured by fist widths and compared side to side.

During the course of the supine examination, any pop in this plane can sometimes be related to a snapping iliopsoas tendon. A fan test (the patient circumducts and rotates the hip in a rotatory fashion) can help delineate the presence of the snapping iliopsoas tendon over the femoral head or the innominate. Often, this diminishes with an abdominal contraction (video). A hula hoop maneuver, in which the patient stands and twists, or a bicycle test (performed in the lateral position), can help distinguish the pop internally from the external pop of coxa sultans externus caused by the subluxing iliotibial band over the greater trochanter.

The FABER test, conventionally known as the Patrick test, is helpful in determining hip versus lumbar complaints (Fig. 1-7). Re-creation of hip pain can be associated with musculotendinous or osseous posterior lateral acetabular incongruence or ligamentous injury. In cases of a coup-contrecoup injury, in which the mechanism of injury is initiated posteriorly, pain will be secondarily referred to anteriorly.

A variety of tests are used for the detection of impingement or intra-articular pathology. The degree of flexion required in this position of adduction—internal rotation depends on the degree of impingement and type and location of the impingement.

For the DIRI test, the patient is in the supine position and instructed to hold the nonaffected leg in flexion beyond 90 degrees, thus establishing a zero pelvic set point and eliminating lumbar lordosis. The examined hip is then brought into 90 degrees of flexion or beyond and is passively taken through a wide arc of adduction and internal rotation (Fig. 1-8). A positive result is noted with re-creation of the complaint pain. DIRI can also be performed in the operating room for direct visualization of femoral neck and acetabular congruence (video).

For the DEXRIT test, the patient is in the supine position and instructed to hold the nonaffected leg in flexion beyond 90 degrees, thus eliminating lumbar lordosis. The hip is then brought into 90 degrees flexion or beyond and dynamically taken through a wide arc of abduction and external rotation (Fig. 1-9). A positive result is noted with re-creation of pain. DEXRIT can be performed intraoperatively for direct visualization of femoral neck and acetabular congruence (video).

Passive abduction and adduction range of motion are assessed in the supine position (see Table 1-3). Palpation of the abdomen is performed and any tenderness is documented (Fig. 1-10). Abdominal tenderness is differentiated from fascial hernia and/or adductor tendinitis. Resisted torso flexion with palpation of the abdomen will differentiate the fascial hernia from other complaints. Palpation of the adductor tubercle with active testing will detect adductor tendonitis. Common physical examination findings associated with athletic pubalgia include inguinal canal tenderness, pubic crest-tubercle tenderness, adductor origin tenderness, pain with resisted sit-ups or hip flexion, and a tender, dilated superficial ring.

Other useful tests may include Tinel's test of the femoral nerve. This test is found to be positive with hip flexion contractures of more than 25 degrees as a result of the proximity of the psoas tendon and femoral nerve. A heel strike is performed by striking the heel abruptly. A positive response is

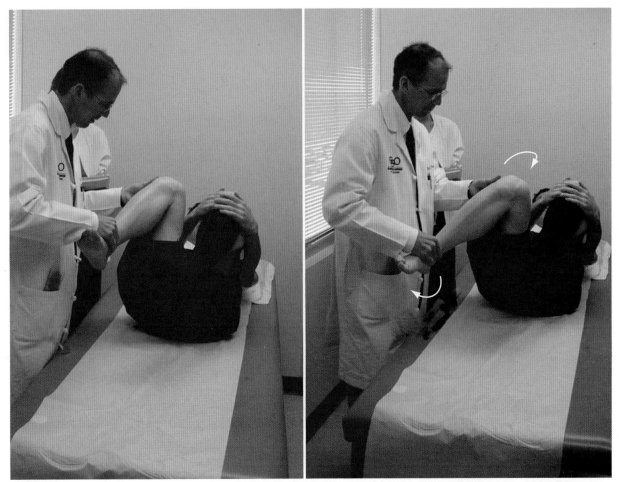

**FIGURE 1-8** Dynamic internal rotatory impingement (DIRI) test. **A,** DIRI begins with the hip at 90 degrees flexion or beyond. **B,** It is then passively taken through a wide arc of adduction and internal rotation (*arrows*) while decreasing flexion to about 80 degrees.

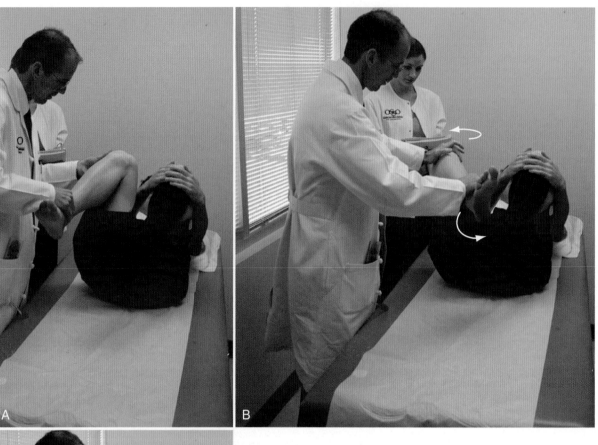

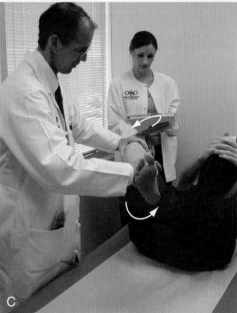

**FIGURE 1-9** The dynamic external rotatory impingement test (DEXRIT). **A,** DEXRIT begins with the hip at 90 degrees flexion or beyond. **B, C,** It is then dynamically taken through a wide arc of abduction and external rotation (*arrows*).

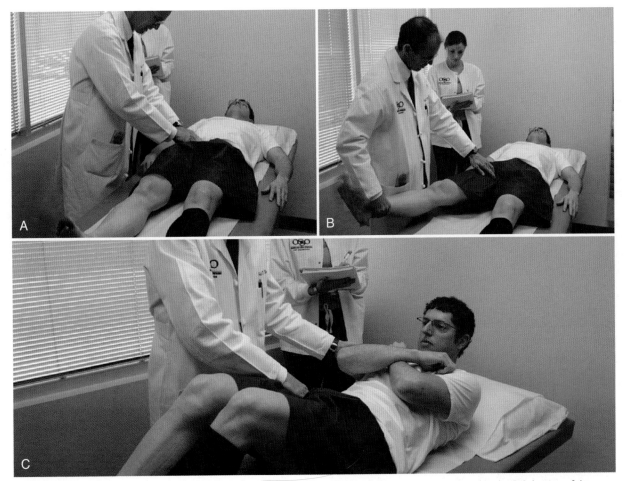

**FIGURE 1-10 A,** Palpation of the abdomen in the relaxed supine position. **B,** Palpation of the adductor tubercle. **C,** Palpation of the abdomen with an abdominal contraction.

indicative of trauma or a stress fracture (Fig. 1-11A). The passive supine rotation test (log roll) involves passive internal and external rotation of the femur, with the leg lying in an extended or slightly flexed position (see Fig. 1-11B). The passive supine rotation test is performed bilaterally and any side to side differences in this maneuver can alert the examiner to the presence of laxity, effusion, or internal derangement. The straight leg raise against resistance test (Stinchfield test) is an assessment of hip flexor and psoas strength and is a sign of an intra-articular problem as the psoas places pressure on the labrum. The patient performs an active straight leg raise, with the knee in extension up to 45 degrees; the examiner's hand is then placed distal to the knee while applying a downward force (see Fig. 1-11C). A positive test is noted with re-creation of the complaint, pain, or weakness.

The importance of multiple examinations is recognized for the detection of intra-articular pathology. Even in the presence of normal internal and external rotation, there is a need for further delineation of the relationships that exist among the musculotendinous, osseous, and ligamentous structures. Tests for impingement can have good specificity and reasonable predictive value for osseous abnormalities; however, no single test is sensitive enough to be used exclusively. Furthermore, the ligamentous contribution to range of motion varies with flexion and rotation.[13]

The posterior rim impingement test can also be performed in the supine position. The patient is positioned at the edge of the examining table so that the examined leg hangs freely at the hip and the patient draws up both legs in to the chest, eliminating lumbar lordosis. The affected leg is then extended off the table, allowing for full extension of the hip, abducted and externally rotated (Fig. 1-12). The posterior rim impingement test takes the hip into extension and assesses the congruence of the posterior acetabular wall and femoral neck. A variation of this test is the lateral rim impingement test (see next section).

### Lateral Examination

The lateral examination (Table 1-5) begins with the patient on the contralateral side and palpating the areas of the suprasacroiliac and sacroiliac (SI) joint, muscles of abduction, and origin of the gluteus maximus as it inserts along the lateral border of the sacrum and the most posterior aspect of the ilium. The next point of palpation is the ischium for detection of avulsions or bursitis. Finally, the piriformis and sciatic

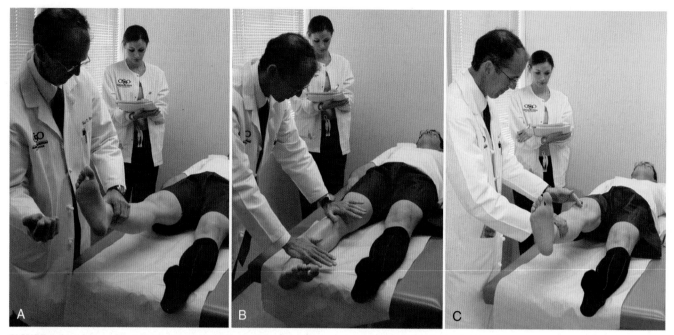

**FIGURE 1-11** Additional tests in the supine position. **A,** The heel strike is performed by striking the heel abruptly. **B,** The passive supine rotation test involves passive internal rotation (shown) and external rotation of the femur, with the leg lying in an extended position. **C,** Straight leg raise against resistance.

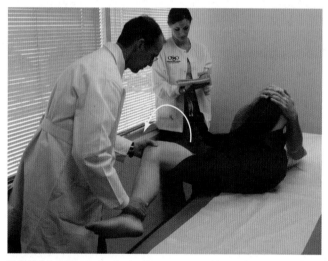

**FIGURE 1-12** Posterior rim impingement test. The patient rests at the edge of the examining table, with the affected leg hanging freely at the hip while holding the contralateral leg in full flexion. The examined leg is then brought into full hip extension, abducted, and externally rotated (*arrow*).

**TABLE 1-5**   Summary of Lateral Examinations and Assessment

| Examination | Assessment and Association |
|---|---|
| Flexion, adduction, internal rotation | Anterior femoroacetabular impingement, torn labrum |
| Lateral rim impingement | Lateral femoroacetabular impingement, torn labrum, instability |
| Tensor fascia lata contracture test (Ober test) | Tensor fascia lata contracture |
| Gluteus medius contracture test (Ober test) | Gluteus medius contracture, tear (decreased strength with knee flexion, suspect tear) |
| Gluteus maximus contracture test | Gluteus maximus contracture, contribution to iliotibial band |
| Palpation | |
|   Greater trochanter | Greater trochanter bursitis, iliotibial band contracture |
|   Sacroiliac joint | Distinguish between hip and back pathology, |
|   Maximus origin | Gluteus maximus origin tendinitis |
|   Ischium | Biceps femoris tendinitis, avulsion fracture, ischial Bursitis |

*See video.*

nerve are palpated for any signs of tenderness, along with the abductor musculature, which includes the glutei (maximus, medius, and minimus) and tensor fascia lata. An active piriformis test is performed by the patient pushing the heel down into the table, abducting and externally rotating the leg against resistance, while the examiner monitors the piriformis (Fig. 1-13). The active piriformis test is similar to Pace's sign, which is pain and weakness on resisted abduction and external rotation of the thigh in the seated position.[14] A set of passive adduction tests (similar to Ober's test) are performed with the leg in three positions (Fig. 1-14)—extension (tensor fascia lata contracture test), neutral (gluteus medius contracture test), and flexion (gluteus maximus contracture test). Gluteus medius tension is assessed by relaxation of the iliotibial band with knee flexion. In this position, the hip should adduct down toward the table. Any restrictions of these motions are recorded. When performing the gluteus maximus contracture test, the shoulder is rotated toward the side of the table, with the hip flexed and knee extended. If adduction cannot occur in this position, the gluteus maximus portion is contracted. The hip should freely be able to come into a full adducted position and any restriction of the gluteus maximus is recognized. The gluteus maximus is balanced with the tensor fascia lata anteriorly. If the hip does not come beyond the midline in the longitudinal axis of the torso, it is graded as a 3+ restriction above torso, 2+ restriction at the midline, and 1+ restriction below. A clear delineation of the exact area of restriction will help direct physical therapy and peritrochanteric treatment options. Strength is assessed with any type of

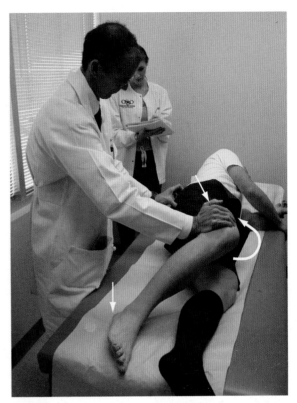

**FIGURE 1-13** Active piriformis test. With the patient in the lateral position, the examiner palpates the piriformis. The patient drives the heel into the examining table, thus initiating external hip rotation while actively abducting and externally rotating against resistance (*arrows*).

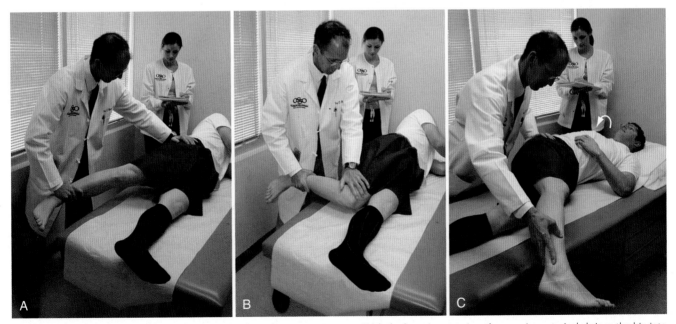

**FIGURE 1-14** Passive adduction tests. **A,** The Tensor fascia lata contracture test: With the knee in extension, the examiner passively brings the hip into extension then adduction. **B,** Gluteus medius contracture test is performed with knee flexion, thus eliminating contribution of the iliotibial band and zero flexion. The examiner passively adducts the hip toward the examination table. **C,** The gluteus maximus contracture test is performed with the ipsilateral shoulder rotated toward the examination table (*arrow*). With the examined leg held in knee extension, the examiner passively brings the hip into flexion and then adduction.

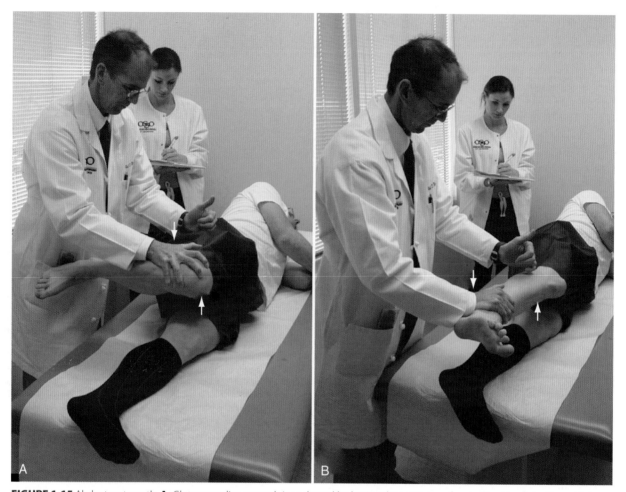

**FIGURE 1-15** Abductor strength. **A,** Gluteus medius strength is evaluated by having the patient perform active hip abduction with knee flexion (*arrows*). **B,** Gluteus maximus strength is evaluated by active hip abduction with knee extension (*arrows*).

lateral-based hip complaint. The gluteus medius strength test is performed with the knee in flexion (Fig. 1-15) to release the iliotibial band contribution.

Next is the passive FADDIR assessment, which is performed in a dynamic manner (Fig. 1-16). The examiner holds the monitoring hand in and about the superior aspect of the hip with the lower leg cradled on the forearm and the knee on the hand. The hip is then brought into flexion, adduction, and internal rotation. Any reproduction of the patient's complaint and the degree of impingement are noted. FADDIR is commonly performed as part of the supine assessment.[15] The difference is the position of the pelvis. The supine position eliminates lumbar lordosis, whereas the lateral tests the normal dynamic pelvic inclination. Pelvic inclination may affect testing and both positions are helpful in evaluation.

The lateral rim impingement Test is performed with the hip passively abducted and externally rotated (Fig. 1-17). The examiner cradles the patient's lower leg with one arm and monitors the hip joint with the opposing hand. The examiner passively brings the affected hip through a wide arc from flexion to extension in continuous abduction while externally rotating the hip. Reproduction of the patient's pain is scored positive. If the feeling of guarding or

instability is present, the test is positive for apprehension, which is not to be confused with coup-contrecoup. The traditional Patrick test is performed in the supine position and is helpful for differentiating hip and back pain. However, when performed in the lateral position, the lateral rim impingement test is useful for the detection of posterior or lateral impingement. Any type of re-creation of a posterior or lateral rim complaint can be precipitated in this position. The lateral rim impingement, FABER, and posterior rim impingement tests all place the hip into positions of posterior and lateral impingement. The lateral rim impingement test establishes a functional lumbar lordosis, with a clear ability to comfortably monitor sites of impingement, which aids in the separation of posterior and lateral points of impingement.

### Prone Examination

The prone examination (Table 1-6) involves palpation of four distinct areas—the supra-SI, SI, gluteus maximus, and spine (facets). Should the pain be identified in the supra-SI joint region in or about the facet, a lumbar hyperextension test can help identify the exact location of suspected pain. If this test is

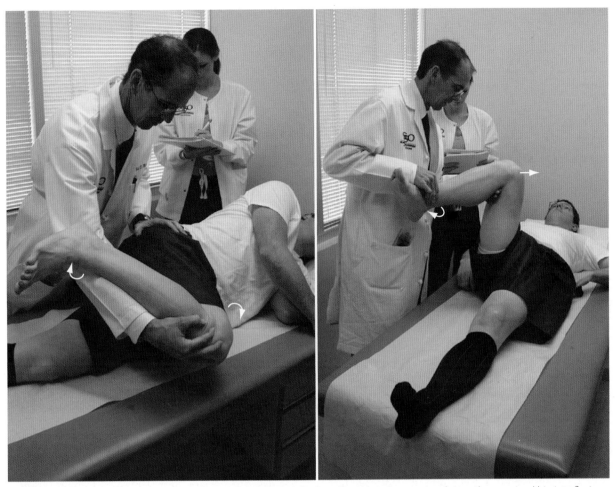

**FIGURE 1-16** Flexion, adduction, internal rotation (FADDIR). **A,** In the lateral position, the examiner brings the examined hip into flexion, adduction, and internal rotation while monitoring the superior aspect of the hip (*arrows*). **B,** FADDIR can also be performed in the supine position (*arrows*).

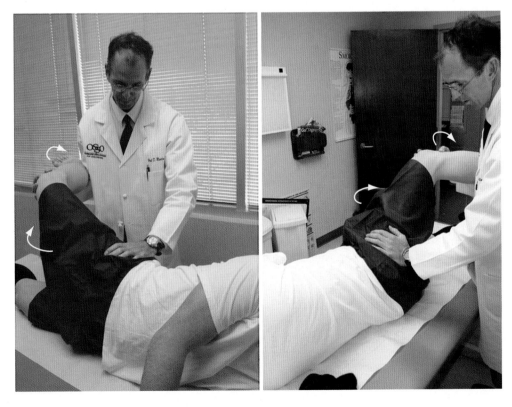

**FIGURE 1-17** Lateral rim impingement test. **A,** Front view. **B,** Rear view. The lateral rim impingement test is performed in the lateral position. The examiner cradles the patient's lower leg with one arm and monitors the hip joint with the opposing hand. The affected hip is passively brought through a wide arc from flexion to extension in continuous abduction while externally rotating the hip (*arrows*).

**TABLE 1-6** Prone Examination

| Examination | Assessment and Association |
|---|---|
| Rectus contracture test (Ely test) | Rectus femoris contracture |
| Femoral anteversion test (Craig test) | Detect increased femoral anteversion or retroversion, ligamentous injury, hyperlaxity |
| Palpation | |
| Supra-SI | Mechanical transverse process ilial conflict |
| SI | Sacroiliitis |
| Gluteus maximus insertion | Gluteus maximus tendinitis |
| Spine | Detect spinal mechanical pathology |
| With lumbar hyperextension | Rule out spine as a prominent or secondary issue |

*See video.*

positive, the patient can then be placed into a supine position, with the knees flexed. If this helps alleviate the pain, the back should be evaluated further.

The femoral anteversion test, traditionally known as Craig's test, will give the examiner an idea of femoral anteversion and retroversion (Fig. 1-18A).[16] With the patient in the prone position, the knee is flexed to 90 degrees and the examiner manually rotates the leg while palpating the greater trochanter. The greater trochanter is positioned so that it protrudes most laterally, thereby placing the femoral head into the center portion of the acetabulum. Femoral version is assessed by noting the angle between the axis of the tibia and an imaginary vertical line. Normally, femoral anteversion is between 10 and 20 degrees.[16] This test will help identify cases of retroversion. If there is a significant difference of internal rotation in the extended and seated (flexed) positions, an osseous versus a ligamentous cause should be differentiated (see Fig. 1-18B). The rectus contracture test (also known as Ely's test) is performed with the patient in the prone position and the lower extremity flexed toward the gluteus maximus (see Fig. 1-18C). Any raise of the pelvis or restriction of hip flexion is indicative of rectus femoris contracture.

### Specific Tests

**McCarthy Test.** This is a maneuver associated with a McCarthy sign, a reproducible pop or click.[8] The McCarthy test is performed with the contralateral leg held in flexion. The examined hip is brought to 90 degrees flexion and then abducted, externally rotated, and extended. The hip is then brought to 90 degrees flexion, adducted, internally rotated, and extended. A positive McCarthy sign is helpful for detecting anterior femoroacetabular impingement or a torn labrum.

**Scour Test.** This is performed in the same manner as DIRI. However, the examiner applies pressure at the knee, thereby increasing pressure at the hip joint, which is helpful for detecting interarticular congruence (video).

**Foveal Distraction Test.** Intra-articular pressure is alleviated by gently pulling the leg away from the body as the patient is in the supine position. The relief of pain or re-creation of pain will help delineate extra- versus intra-articular pathology (video).

**Bicycle Test.** This is performed with the patient in the lateral position. The motion of a bicycle pedaling pattern is re-created as the examiner monitors the iliotibial band for the detection of coxa sultans externus (video).

**Fulcrum Test.** The examiner's knee is placed under the patient's knee, acting as the fulcrum. The patient then performs a straight leg test against resistance.

**Seated Piriformis Stretch Test – (Figure 1-19).** The seated position offers a stable and reproducible platform with the hip at 90° of flexion. The examiner extends the knee and passively moves the flexed hip into adduction with internal rotation while palpating 1cm lateral to the ischium (middle finger) and proximally at the sciatic notch (index finger). A positive test is the recreation of the posterior pain. Freiberg has described sciatic nerve entrapment by the piriformis[17] and may be entrapped in other areas which is best described as Deep Gluteal Syndrome[18]. Pain in the buttock may be caused from entrapment of the sciatic nerve by the piriformis muscle, hamstring, obturator internus/gemelli complex, or scar tissue. Piriformis syndrome is often due to scarring between the sciatic nerve and external rotators[19]. The inferior gluteal nerve, inferior gluteal artery and sciatic nerve may be scarred into the hamstring tendons due to trauma or avulsion of the hamstring[20]. Irritation of the structures of the obturator internus/gemelli complex are commonly overlooked in association with back pain and may cause sciatica-like pain[21,22]. The use of palpation of the involved anatomy along with a physical exam that includes the Straight Leg Raise Test, the Seated Piriformis Stretch Test, and Pace's test will aid in the differential diagnosis of deep gluteal syndrome.

**Abduction, Extension, External Rotation Test.** The abduction, extension, external rotation (ABDEER) test is performed in the lateral position with the affected leg passively brought into abduction, extension, and external rotation as forward pressure is applied to the posterior aspect of the hip. Re-creation of the patient's pain is a positive test. As with the apprehension test performed on the shoulder, ABDEER is helpful for the detection of any type of anterior capsular laxity or injury. Of note, current research suggests that this position specifically releases the teres ligament.

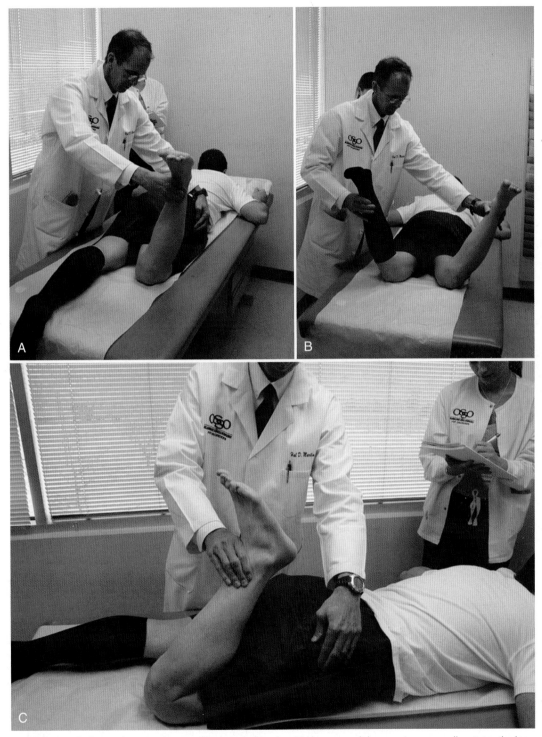

**FIGURE 1-18 A,** Femoral anteversion test. The knee is flexed to 90 degrees and the examiner manually rotates the leg while palpating the greater trochanter. The examiner positions the greater trochanter so that it protrudes most laterally, noting the angle between the axis of the tibia and an imaginary vertical line. **B,** Internal rotation in the extended position. Note any differences from the seated flexed position. **C,** Rectus contracture test. The lower extremity is flexed toward the gluteus maximus. Any raise of the pelvis or restriction of hip flexion motion is indicative of rectus femoris contracture.

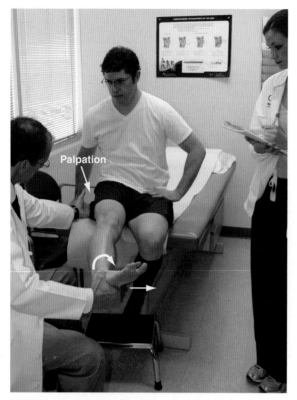

**FIGURE 1-19** Seated Piriformis Stretch Test. The patient is in the seated position with knee extension. The examiner passively moves the flexed hip into adduction with internal rotation while palpating 1cm lateral to the ischium (middle finger) and proximally at the sciatic notch (index finger).

**Dynamic Trendelenburg Test.**   With the patient in a single-leg stance, the examiner applies a slight force or shove to the patient's shoulder. By introducing this dynamic component to single-leg standing, subtle signs of strength or proprioception deficits may be elicited (video).

**Supine Abduction External Rotation Test.**   Performed in the supine position, the hip is taken into abduction and external rotation at varying degrees of flexion to extension to distinguish internal derangements, laxity, or impingement (video).

**Resisted Sit-up Test.**   The athletic hernia is described as a condition of a weakened posterior wall of the inguinal canal, which results in chronic pain in the groin that may refer to other surrounding areas and is exacerbated with activity.[23] Although the term *hernia* is associated with a bulge, it is common that no true hernia is present following laparoscopic repair. Diagnosis of the athletic hernia may be difficult because this pain may mimic the pain associated with hip pathologies. The typical athletic hernia symptoms consist of dull pain in the area of the groin that may radiate to the perineum and inner thigh or across the midline.[23] Common physical examination findings include inguinal canal tenderness, pubic crest-tubercle tenderness, adductor origin tenderness, pain

with resisted sit-ups or hip flexion, and a tender, dilated, superficial ring.[23]

**Pudendal Nerve Block Test.**   Four clinical features must be present for a diagnosis of pudendal nerve entrapment according to the Nantes criteria.[24] These include pain in the urogenital area that is increased with sitting and that does not wake the patient at night, as well as loss of sensation of the genitalia. If these essential criteria are met, a diagnostic anesthetic pudendal nerve block should be carried out; relief of symptoms strongly supports the diagnosis.

To summarize, the physical examination of the hip encompasses examination of the hip, back, and lower extremities, as well as the abdominal, vascular, and neuromuscular systems. In the evaluation of the hip, it is necessary also to examine joints above and below the hip. Record a complete patient history, perform physical examination tests properly and consistently, and be aware of concomitant pathologies. By performing the physical examination of the hip as described, the surgeon will have a well-established reference grid leading to an accurate diagnosis, be able to follow the patient before and after treatment accurately, distinguish osseous, ligamentous, and musculotendinous pathology, and understand which radiographic tests will be required for a comprehensive diagnosis and treatment recommendations.

## RADIOGRAPHIC ANALYSES

### Evaluation by Standing Anteroposterior and Frog-Leg Lateral Views

To evaluate patients who present with hip pain fully, the following radiographic views are obtained—a standing and supine anteroposterior (AP) pelvic and frog-leg lateral view.[25] Each radiographic view is critical in the diagnostic evaluation and treatment of structural abnormalities. There are a number of other radiographic views available, such as cross-table lateral,[26] false profile,[27,28] and 45- and 90-degree Dunn views,[29] which physicians may prefer on an individual basis.[30]

The standing AP radiograph (Fig. 1-20) is made with the patient standing with the feet in neutral rotation and shoulder width apart to resemble the natural biomechanical stance as related to gait. The feet may also be placed parallel to each other, with enough internal rotation for the feet to touch.[31] The x-ray tube-to-film distance should be 120 cm, with the crosshairs centered on the midpoint between the superior border of the pubic symphysis and a line drawn connecting the anterior superior iliac spines (ASISs).[30] The coccyx should be centered in line with the pubic symphysis, and the iliac wings, obturator foramina, and radiographic teardrops should be symmetrical in appearance. If pelvic inclination is appropriate, a 1- to 3-cm gap should be seen between the superior border of the pubic symphysis and the tip of the coccyx.[32] This particular radiograph is used because acetabular roof obliquity, center edge angle, and minimum joint space width may vary between weight-bearing and supine positions.[33] Ensuring symmetry is critical to the interpretation of radiographic findings.

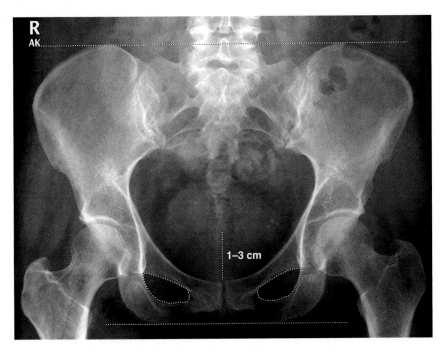

**FIGURE 1-20** The standing AP radiograph is made with the patient standing with the feet in neutral rotation and shoulder width apart in stance. The coccyx should be centered in line with the pubic symphysis, and the iliac wings, obturator foramina, and radiographic teardrops should be symmetrical in appearance. If pelvic inclination is appropriate, a 1- to 3-cm gap should be seen between the superior border of the pubic symphysis and the tip of the coccyx.

The standing AP radiograph will assess the following: (1) functional leg length inequalities; (2) neck shaft angle (NSA); (3) femoral neck trabecular patterns; (4) lateral and anterior center edge angles; (5) acetabular inclination; (6) joint space width; (7) lateralization; (8) head sphericity; (9) acetabular cup depth; and (10) anterior and posterior wall orientation (Fig. 1-21).

## Pathologic Definitions of Radiographic Findings

**Functional Leg Lengths.** These should be considered when a patient presents with hip-related symptoms. The total length of one leg should be compared with the contralateral leg length by examining the superior border of the iliac crests. A

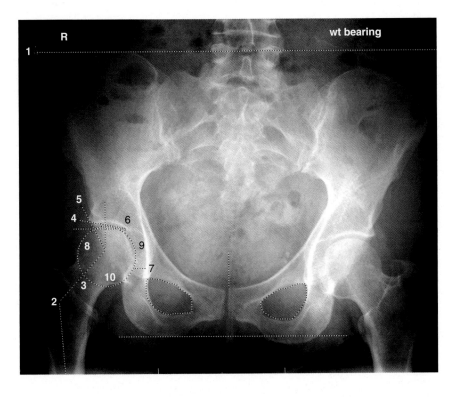

**FIGURE 1-21** The standing AP radiograph will assess 1 functional leg length inequalities, 2 neck shaft angle, 3 femoral neck trabecular patterns, 4 acetabular inclination, 5 lateral center edge angles, 6 joint space width, 7 lateralization, 8 head sphericity, 9 acetabular cup depth, and 10 anterior and posterior wall orientation.

leg length discrepancy (LLD) of more than 2.0 cm can have an adverse effect on the kinematic function of the hip.[34] The difference in functional leg lengths is usually a combination of structural differences of the long bones, hemipelvis, or spine.

**Neck Shaft Angle.**   The NSA dictates the load transfer from the femur to the acetabulum. It is the angle formed by the longitudinal axes of the femoral neck and the proximal femoral diaphyseal axis.[35] One line is drawn parallel to the midpoint of the femoral neck and one is drawn parallel to the midpoint of the femoral shaft. The angle formed represents the NSA. Normal values range from 125 to 140 degrees. If the NSA is more than 140 degrees, it is classified as coxa valgus; if less than 125 degrees, it is classified as coxa varus. The normal neck shaft angle produces the lowest stress on the femoral neck and acetabulum because of the orientation of an optimal lever arm that produces a mechanical advantage for biomechanical function.

**Trabecular Pattern.**   This is examined radiographically to visualize the influence of the neck shaft angle on the compressive and tensile forces within the femoral neck. In cases of coxa varus, tensile trabeculae are more prominent, whereas in cases of coxa valgus, compressive trabeculae are more prominent (Fig. 1-22).[36]

**Lateral Center Edge Angles.**   Lateral center edge angles (LCAs) are used to assess the degree of acetabular coverage of the femoral head. The lateral center edge angle is formed by a line drawn parallel to the longitudinal pelvic axis and a line connecting the center of the femoral head with the lateral edge of the acetabulum.[37] Normal values range from 22 to 42 degrees

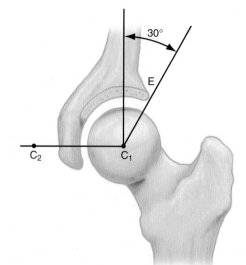

**FIGURE 1-23** Center edge (CE) angle. The vertical line is perpendicular to the horizontal line extending from the center of each femoral head ($C_1$ and $C_2$). The E (edge) point is the most lateral point of the acetabulum. The CE angle is measured between the vertical and the line passing through $C_1$ or $C_2$ and E. *(Redrawn from Delaunay S, Dussault RG, Kaplan PA, Alford BA. Radiographic measurements of dysplastic adult hips. Skeletal Radiol. 1997;26:75-81.)*

in adults, although values less than 26 degrees may indicate inadequate coverage of the femoral head (Fig. 1-23).[34,38]

**Anterior Center Edge Angles.**   Anterior center edge angles (ACEs) are assessed from a false profile view and are determined if there is dysplasia to help locate acetabular overcoverage.[26,39,40] The false profile view is performed with the patient standing with the affected hip against the cassette and pelvis

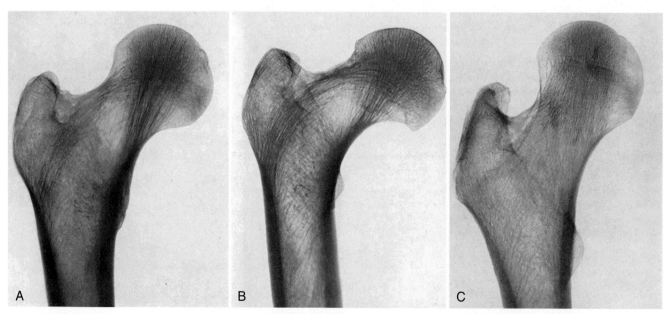

**FIGURE 1-22 A,** The trabecular pattern is examined radiographically to visualize the influence of the neck shaft angle on the compressive and tensile forces within the femoral neck. This pattern is normal. In cases of coxa varus **(B)**, tensile trabeculae are more prominent, whereas in cases of coxa valgus **(C)**, compressive trabeculae are more prominent. *(From Pauwels F. Biomechanics of the Normal and Diseased Hip. New York: Springer-Verlag; 1976.)*

rotated 65 degrees in relation to the wall stand. The foot on the same side as the affected hip is placed parallel to the cassette. The central beam is centered on the femoral head with a tube-to-film distance of 120 cm. A vertical line and a line connecting the center of the femoral head with the anterior edge of the acetabulum form the ACE. In consideration for intertrochanteric osteotomy (ITO) and periacetabular osteotomy (PAO), an abducted internal rotation radiograph allows for the examination of the centralization of the femoral head with improved acetabular coverage.

**Acetabular Inclination.** This is the angle (Tonnis angle of inclination)[35] formed by a horizontal line and a tangent from the lowest point of the sclerotic zone of the acetabular roof to the lateral edge of the acetabulum (Fig. 1-24). Three classifications are used for acetabular inclination[30,41]:

1. Normal = Tonnis angle of 0 to 10 degrees
2. Increased = Tonnis angle > 10 degrees, subject to structural instability
3. Decreased = Tonnis angle < 0 degrees, subject to pincer-type femoroacetabular impingement (FAI)

**Joint Space Width.** This is measured as the shortest distance between the femoral head surface and acetabulum, centrally and laterally, at the weight-bearing sclerotic zone (see Fig. 1-24). Joint space width is examined using the standing AP

radiograph because the effects of position influence the joint space observed.[42] Any evidence of joint space narrowing can be classified using the Tonnis grade for osteoarthritis.[35] The Tonnis grade[41] for osteoarthritis can be correlated using all radiographic views, but the final grade is determined on the basis of the single view with the highest overall degree of osteoarthritic change.[30]

**Hip Center Position.** If the medial aspect of the femoral head is more than 10 mm from the ilioischial line, the hip is classified as lateralized and nonlateralized if the medial aspect of the femoral head is within a 10-mm margin from the ilioischial line. Comparisons from side to side may help determine any amount of lateralization (see Fig. 1-24).

**Head Sphericity.** This should be assessed on standing AP and frog-leg lateral radiographs because a patient may have an apparently spherical head on the AP view, but not on the lateral view. The femoral head is classified as spherical if the epiphysis does not extend beyond the margin of a reference circle by more than 2 mm and is classified as aspherical if it extends beyond this 2-mm margin (see Fig. 1-24).[43,44]

**Acetabular Cup Depth.** The relationship of the floor of the fossa acetabuli and femoral head are evaluated relative to the ilioischial line. If the floor of the fossa acetabuli touches or is medial to the ilioischial line, or the posterior wall extends

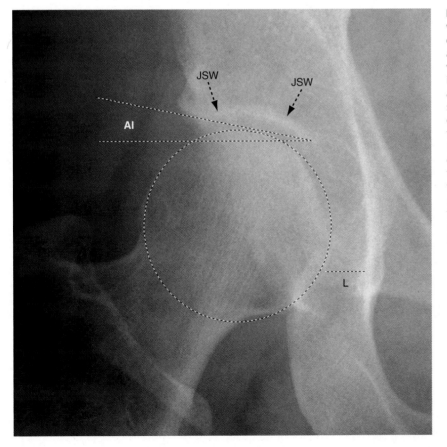

**FIGURE 1-24** Standing AP radiograph. Joint space width (JSW; *arrows*) is measured as the shortest distance between the femoral head surface and acetabulum, both centrally and laterally, at the weight-bearing sclerotic zone. The acetabular index (AI) is the angle formed by a horizontal line and a tangent from the lowest point of the sclerotic zone of the acetabular roof to the lateral edge of the acetabulum. If the medial aspect of the femoral head is >10 mm from the ilioischial line, the hip is classified as lateralized (L); it is classified as nonlateralized if the medial aspect of the femoral head is within a 10-mm margin from the ilioischial line. The femoral head is classified as spherical if the epiphysis does not extend beyond the margin of a reference circle by more than 2 mm and aspherical if it does extend beyond this 2-mm margin.

lateral to the center axis of rotation, the hip is classified as coxa profunda. If the medial aspect of the femoral head is medial to the ilioischial line, the head is classified as protrusio.[45] Also, the inner acetabular wall thickness, medial wall shape, and inferior cup orientation should be recognized.

**Acetabular Version.** Acetabula can be classified as anteverted or retroverted based on the presence or absence of a crossover sign (Fig. 1-25).[46] The acetabulum is classified as anteverted if the line of the anterior aspect of the rim does not cross the line of the posterior aspect of the rim before reaching the lateral aspect of the sourcil. If the anterior aspect of the rim does cross the line of the posterior aspect of the rim before reaching the lateral edge of the sourcil, the acetabulum is classified as retroverted. It is important to note that true acetabular retroversion is associated with a deficient posterior wall,[46] whereas a hip with a crossover sign but no posterior wall deficiency refers to anterior overcoverage—cranial acetabular retroversion or anterior focal acetabular retroversion.[30,47] Both standing and supine AP radiographs should be used to determine anterior and posterior wall inclination, again ensuring good quality because of the possibility of overinterpreting the incidence of retroversion.[33]

**Frog-Leg Lateral Radiograph.** This allows for the assessment of another view of medial and lateral joint space width, femoral head sphericity, congruency, head-neck offset, alpha angle, and bone morphology (Fig. 1-26). The frog-leg lateral radiograph should be taken with the patient supine, the affected limb flexed at the knee approximately 30 to 40 degrees, and the hip abducted to 45 degrees . The heel should rest against the medial aspect of the contralateral knee. The cassette is placed so that the top of the film rests at the ASIS and the crosshairs directed midway between the ASIS and pubic symphysis. The x-ray tube-to-film distance should be approximately 102 cm. This particular orientation is used because it is easily reproducible in the operating room and allows for a consistent radiographic view of the head-neck junction offset during the pre- and intraoperative radiographic examination.

**Head-Neck Offset.** This is assessed from the frog-leg lateral radiograph and is classified based on the gross appearance of the relationship between the radius curvatures of the anterior aspect of the femoral head with the posterior aspect of the head neck junction.[43] The head-neck offset is classified as symmetrical if the anterior and posterior concavities are grossly symmetrical. If the anterior concavity has a radius of curvature greater than that at the posterior aspect of the head-neck (H-N) junction, it is classified as having a moderate decrease in H-N offset. If the anterior aspect has a convexity, as opposed to a concavity, the head-neck junction is classified as having a prominence (CAM-type FAI).[43]

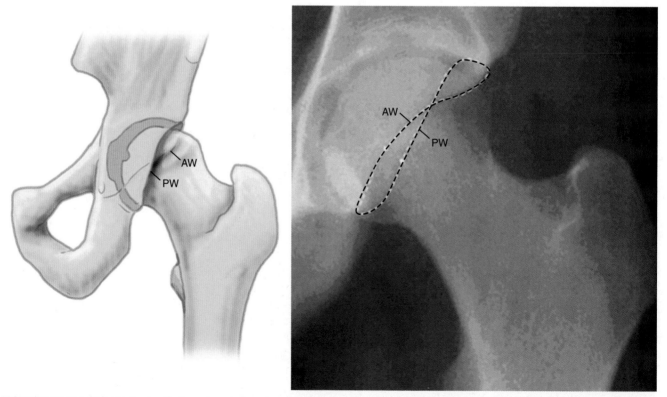

**FIGURE 1-25** Acetabula can be classified as anteverted or retroverted based on the presence or absence of a crossover of the anterior wall (AW) and posterior wall (PW). The inner acetabular wall thickness, medial wall shape, and inferior cup orientation should be recognized. *(From Tannast M, Siebenrock KA, Anderson SE. Femoroacetabular impingement: radiographic diagnosis—what the radiologist should know. AJR Am J Roentgenol. 2007;188:1540-1552)*

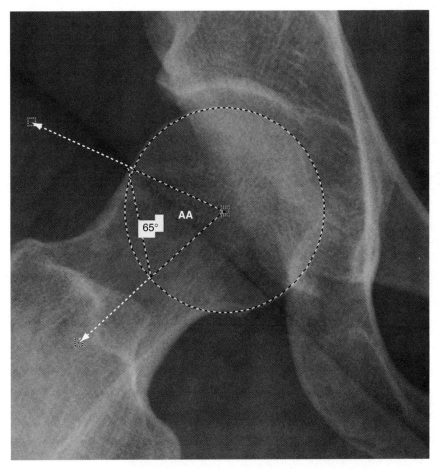

**FIGURE 1-26** The 30-degree frog-leg lateral radiograph allows for the assessment of another view of medial and lateral joint space width, femoral head sphericity, congruency, head-neck offset, and alpha angle (AA), as well as bone morphology. The femoral head is classified as spherical if the epiphysis does not extend beyond the margin of a reference circle by more than 2 mm and aspherical if it does extend beyond this 2-mm margin. A prominence is shown on the femoral neck where the top line intersects the reference circle.

**Alpha Angle.** This is calculated by drawing a line from the center of the femoral head to the point on the anterolateral aspect of the head-neck junction where the radius of the femoral head deviates from the more central femoral head radius in the acetabulum, or where a prominence starts, and a line drawn through the center of the femoral neck to the center of the femoral head (see Fig. 1-26). Values of more than 42 degrees are suggestive of head-neck offset deformity,[30] but are dependent on acetabular femoral congruency.[34]

## Cross-Sectional Imaging Techniques

The use of cross-sectional imaging (Fig. 1-27) is essential for the evaluation of patients for intra- and extra-articular pathology. Imaging protocols such as magnetic resonance imaging (MRI), magnetic resonance arthrography (MRA),[48] multidetector computed tomography (MDCT),[34] and computed tomography (CT)[49] allow for the assessment of basic structural torsional alignment that give rise to or predispose patients to certain types of pathology such as FAI, acetabular tears, or articular damage.

The McKibbin instability index can be calculated from MRI scans and is based on the assumption that the effects of femoral and acetabular anteversion may be additive or may offset each other. It is calculated as the sum of the angles of femoral and acetabular anteversion, with an index

of 60 denoting severe instability. Deviation is classified as ranging from grade −3, for a low instability index of less than 20, to grade +3, for a high instability index of more than 50.[50] For this technique, the feet should be pointing straight ahead and held in place by a brace or tape to ensure that the geometric relationship of the acetabulum and femur are properly evaluated.

MDCT (see Fig. 1-27) is useful for assessing osseous structures and surrounding soft tissues of the hip and acetabulum and provides data that have the same resolution in the longitudinal axis ($z$ axis) as in the $x$ or $y$ axis.[34] This relationship is important to understand because of the potential not only to detect anatomic derangements that may allow movements that create primary pathology, but also to correct the underlying anatomic abnormalities that may predispose the patient to recurrent or persistent pathology.

MRA (Figs. 1-28 and 1-29) provides assistance in the evaluation of intra-articular pathology of the hip. The detection of acetabular labral tears may assist in confirming a decision for arthroscopic surgery and has been reported to have a positive predictive value of 93%.[51] MRA may also be helpful in the evaluation of mild osseous abnormalities, such as acetabular retroversion and reduced head-neck offset, the integrity of the acetabular labrum, and articular cartilage surface. The ability to detect these subtle abnormalities accurately may be affected by the technique and experience of the radiologist

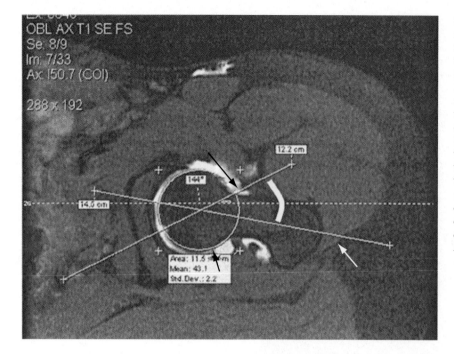

**FIGURE 1-27** MDCT is useful for assessing osseous structures and surrounding soft tissues of the hip and acetabulum. It provides data that have the same resolution in the longitudinal axis (*z* axis) as in the *x* or *y* axis. Oblique axial T1-weighted MR image shows the alpha angle (*white arc*), which is calculated by drawing a line down the center of the femoral head and neck (*white arrow*) and a circle around the periphery of the femoral head (*black arrowhead*). A second line is drawn from the femoral head center, where the anterior osseous femur intersects the circle drawn around the femoral head (*black arrow*). Normal values are <55 degrees. *(From Beall DP, Martin HD, Mintz DN, et al. Anatomic and structural evaluation of the hip: a cross-sectional imaging technique combining anatomic and biomechanical evaluations.* Clin Imaging. *2008; 32:372-381.)*

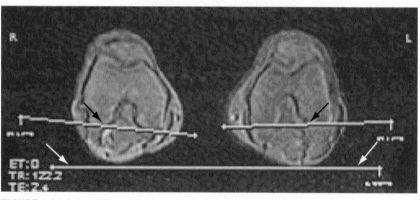

**FIGURE 1-28** Axial gradient echo MR image of the knees taken from a tri-plane localizer sequence shows the coronal reference line (*white arrows*) and the posterior intercondylar line (*white line with black shadowing indicated by the black arrows*). The amount of internal or external rotation is then compared with the coronal reference line and the overall amount of femoral version is calculated. For example, if the proximal femur shows 3 degrees of external rotation and the distal femur shows 15 degrees of internal rotation, the amount of anteversion of the femur is 18 degrees (from 3 degrees external rotation proximally to 15 degrees of internal rotation distally). Foot rotation must be controlled by bracing or taping between the two images. *(From Beall DP, Martin HD, Mintz DN, et al. Anatomic and structural evaluation of the hip: a cross-sectional imaging technique combining anatomic and biomechanical evaluations.* Clin Imaging. *2008;32:372-381.)*

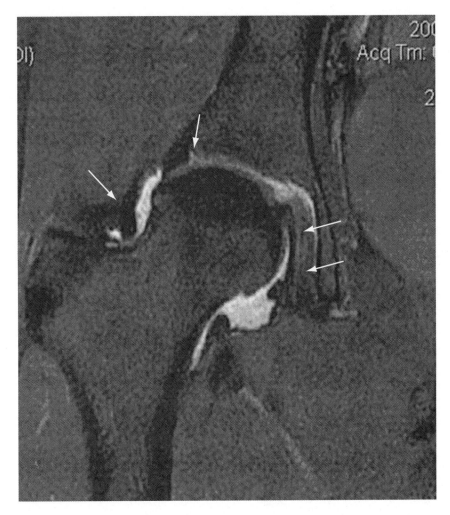

**FIGURE 1-29** Coronal T2-weighted MRI scan with fat saturation taken after direct arthrographic injection with gadolinium shows thickening of the ligamentum teres femoris (*large white arrows*) and of the ligamentous junction between the ligamentum orbicularis and the iliofemoral ligament (*white arrowhead*). The femoral head is slightly displaced laterally in relation to the lateral osseous edge of the acetabulum (*small white arrow*), resulting in some uncovering of the lateral femoral head. *(From Beall DP, Martin HD, Mintz DN, et al. Anatomic and structural evaluation of the hip: a cross-sectional imaging technique combining anatomic and biomechanical evaluations.* Clin Imaging. *2008;32:372-381.)*

and by the quality of scanner used for imaging. Research using delayed gadolinium-enhanced magnetic resonance imaging of cartilage (dGEMRIC), which measures the loss of glycosaminoglycans in the early stages of arthritis, has demonstrated that dGEMRIC can detect early stages of osteoarthritis caused by hip dysplasia and femoroacetabular impingement.[52]

---

**PEARLS & PITFALLS**

**PEARLS**

1. Use a structured physical examination and standardized technique.
2. Ensure quality standardized AP and lateral radiographic examinations.
3. Understand the torsional alignment of femur and acetabulum by MRI or CT techniques.
4. Perform specific additional ancillary tests, as needed.
5. Prior to surgical consideration note internal rotation, external rotation, femoral version, acetabular version, neck shaft angle, acetabular index, center edge, and functional score (HHS).

**PITFALLS**

1. Poor quality physical or radiographic exams lead to misinterpretations.

---

2. Using only two views to analyze dynamic three-planar hip pathology is incomplete. The third axis must be evaluated to understand the complexity of hip biomechanics.
3. Variations in terminology and technique for descriptive tests lead to communication and testing difficulties.

---

## SUMMARY AND CONCLUSIONS

As our understanding of hip pathology advances, the physical examination of the hip continues to evolve. To understand the findings fully, one must be familiar with the anatomy and biomechanics of the hip joint. The use of a formalized, reproducible physical examination will help identify and distinguish osseous, musculotendinous, and ligamentous abnormalities and their comorbidities in a timely fashion (Fig. 1-30). Radiographs and cross-sectional imaging techniques, together with a standardized physical examination, will aid in the preoperative, intraoperative, and postoperative assessment of the hip. The physical examination of the hip is also used as a guide to monitor physical therapy and postoperative rehabilitation. This chapter has introduced a framework of discussion regarding clinically and biomechanically relevant physical examinations.

**PHYSICAL EXAMINATION:**  HT:_____  WT:_____  T:_____  R:_____  P:_____  BP:_____

**Gait/Posture:**

- Shoulder height:          Equal    Not equal
- Iliac crest height:        Equal    Not equal
- Active forward bend:    _____ Degrees
- Spine:        straight
                scoliosis:        structural           non-structural
- Recurvatum: thumb test     elbows          knees        >5 degrees
- Lordosis:     normal          increased       paravertebral muscle spasms
- Gait:         normal          antalgic        abductor deficient (Trendelenburg)
                pelvic wink     arm swing       short stride length         short stance phase

        Foot progression angle:     external        neutral        hyperpronation
- Single leg stance phase test (Trendelenburg Test):       R_____               L_____

**Seated Examination:**

- Neurologic findings:
    Motor:              _____
    Sensory:            _____
    DTR:            Achilles_____         Patella_____
- Circulation:           DP_____         PT_____
- Skin inspection:       _____
- Lymphatic:             lymphedema      no lymphedema        pitting edema: 1+  2+
- Straight leg raise:    R_____    L_____
- Range of motion:      Internal rotation:        External rotation:
                         R_____    L_____        R_____    L_____

**Supine Examination:**

- Leg lengths:      R___cm        L___cm          equal/not equal
- ROM:              Right leg                       Left leg

    Flexion:        80  100  110  120  130  140     80  100  110  120  130  140
    Abduction:      10   20   30   45   50          10   20   30   45   50
    Adduction:       0   10   20   30                0   10   20   30

- Hip flexion contracture test (Thomas Test):           R  +  −              L  +  −
    FADDIR:                                             R  +  −              L  +  −
- DIRI:                                                 R  +  −              L  +  −
- DEXRIT:                                               R  +  −              L  +  −
    Posterior rim impingement test:                     R  +  −              L  +  −
        Apprehension sign:                              R  +  −              L  +  −
- Abdomen:                                              Tender               Non-tender
- Adductor tubercle:                                    Tender               Non-tender
- Palpation pubic symphysis/Adductor                    Tender               Non-tender
- Tinels − femoral nerve                                R  +  −              L  +  −
- FABER (Patrick Test):                                 R  +  −              L  +  −
- Straight leg raise against resistance (Stitchfield Test):   R  +  −         L  +  −
- Passive supine rotation test (Log Roll Test):         R  +  −              L  +  −
- Heel strike:                                          R  +  −              L  +  −

**Lateral Examination:**

- Palpation:
    SI joint                    Tender      Non-tender
    Ischium                     Tender      Non-tender
    Greater trochanter          Tender      Non-tender
    ASIS                        Tender      Non-tender
    Piriformis                  Tender      Non-tender
    Tinels − sciatic nerve
    G. Max insertion into ITB   Tender      Non-tender
    Sciatic nerve               Tender      Non-tender
    Gluteus medius              Tender      Non-tender
    Abductor strength:      Straight leg_____   Gluteus max_____   Gluteus medius_____
- Tensor fascia lata contracture test:      Grade (1–3)_____
- Gluteus medius contracture test:          Grade (1–3)_____
- Gluteus maximus contracture test:         Grade (1–3)_____
- Lateral rim impingement test:             R  +  −        L  +  −
- FADDIR test:                              R  +  −        L  +  −

**FIGURE 1-30** Physical examination of the hip—intake form.                    *Continued*

**Prone Examination:**
- Rectus contracture test (Ely's Test):   R  +  –      L  +  –
- Femoral anteversion test (Craig's Test): _____ degrees anteversion
- Palpation:
  - Spinous processes
  - SI joints                            +  –
  - Bursae ischium                     R  +  –      L  +  –

**Specific Tests**

Philippon Internal Rotation Test          Seated Piriformis Stretch Test
McCarthy's Sign                           Pace Sign
Scours                                    ABDEER
Foveal distraction                        Dynamic Trendelenberg
Bicycle                                   Supine abduction external rotation
Fulcrum

**RADIOLOGY REVIEW:**

<u>Standing A/P</u>
1. Leg lengths:                Right long        Left long
2. Neck shaft angle:           _____ degrees
3. Trabecular pattern:         Normal            Compression dominance
4. Center edge angle:          _____ degrees
5. Acetabular inclination:     _____ degrees
   Acetabular dome shape:      I       II        III  A.  B.  C.
6. Joint space width:
   Central:                    0 mm  2 mm  3 mm  4 mm  5 mm
   Lateral:                    0 mm  2 mm  3 mm  4 mm  5 mm
7. Lateralization:             _____ mm
8. Head sphericity:            Less than 2 mm    Greater than 2 mm
9. Acetabular cup depth:       Profunda          Protrusio
10. Anterior posterior wall orientation:  Anteversion  Retroversion  High retroversion

Others:
Sclerosis          Herniation pit          Thin inner table
Osteophytes        Retained hardware       Teres insertion

<u>Lateral</u>
Alpha angle: ____ degrees          Head sphericity: <2 mm  >2 mm
Herniation pit                     Anterior margin osteophytes

<u>Biometrics</u>
Alpha angle:          Femoral version:          Acetabular version:
____ degrees          ____ degrees              ____ degrees

<u>MRI/Arthrogram</u>
Labrum:                    Torn    Normal
Tear type:                 Grade _____
Location:                  Anterior    Superior    Lateral    Posterior
Iliopsoas tendon shape     IT band
Iliofemoral ligament on axial    Os acetabuli
Bone edema                 Cyst
AVN:  Grade _____
Ligamentum teres

**FIGURE 1-30, cont'd**

## ACKNOWLEDGMENTS

I would like to thank Shea A. Shears, Aaron M. Smathers, Ian J. Palmer, and all the members of the MAHORN (Multicenter Arthroscopy of the Hip Outcomes Research Network) Group who were instrumental in the development of this chapter.

## REFERENCES

1. Philippon M, Schenker M, Briggs K, Kuppersmith D. Femoroacetabular impingement in 45 professional athletes: associated pathologies and return to sport following arthroscopic decompression. *Knee Surg Sports Traumatol Arthrosc.* 2007; 15: 908-914.
2. Bellamy N, Buchanan WW, Goldsmith CH, et al. Validation study of WOMAC: a health status instrument for measuring clinically important patient relevant outcomes to antirheumatic drug therapy in patients with osteoarthritis of the hip or knee. *J Rheumatol.* 1988; 15:1833-1840.
3. Martin RL, Philippon MJ. Evidence of reliability and responsiveness for the hip outcome score. *Arthroscopy.* 2008; 24:676-682.
4. Scopp JM, Moorman CT 3rd. The assessment of athletic hip injury. *Clin Sports Med.* 2001; 20:647-659.
5. DeAngelis NA, Busconi BD. Assessment and differential diagnosis of the painful hip. *Clin Orthop Relat Res.* 2003;(406):11-18.
6. Kujala UM, Kaprio J, Sarna S. Osteoarthritis of weight bearing joints of lower limbs in former elite male athletes. *BMJ.* 1994; 308:231-234.
7. Boyd KT, Peirce NS, Batt ME. Common hip injuries in sport. *Sports Med.* 1997; 24:273-288.

8. Byrd JWT. Physical examination. In: Byrd JWT, ed. *Operative Hip Arthroscopy.* New York: Springer; 2005:36-50.

9. Martin HD. Clinical examination of the hip. *Oper Tech Orthop.* 2005; 15:177-181.

10. Braly BA, Beall DP, Martin HD. Clinical examination of the athletic hip. *Clin Sports Med.* 2006; 25:199-210.

11. Torry MR, Schenker ML, Martin HD, et al. Neuromuscular hip biomechanics and pathology in the athlete. *Clin Sports Med.* 2006; 25:179-197.

12. Perry J. *Gait Analysis: Normal and Pathological Function.* Thorofare, NJ: Slack; 1992.

13. Martin HD, Savage A, Braly BA, et al. The function of the hip capsular ligaments: a quantitative report. *Arthroscopy.* 2008; 24: 188-195.

14. Pace JB, Nagle D. Piriform syndrome. *West J Med.*1976;124: 435-439.

15. Klaue K, Durnin CW, Ganz R. The acetabular rim syndrome. A clinical presentation of dysplasia of the hip. *J Bone Joint Surg Br.*1991;73:423-429.

16. Reider B, Martel J. Pelvis, hip and thigh. In: Reider B, Martel J, eds. *The Orthopedic Physical Examination.* Philadelphia: WB Saunders; 1999:159-199.

17. Freiberg A. Sciatic pain and its relief by operations on muscle and fascia. *Arch Surg.* 1937; 34:337-350.

18. McCrory P, Bell S. Nerve entrapment syndromes as a cause of pain in the hip, groin and buttock. *Sports Med.* 1999; 27:261-274.

19. Benson ER, Schutzer SF. Posttraumatic piriformis syndrome: diagnosis and results of operative treatment. *J Bone Joint Surg Am.*1999;81:941-949.

20. Miller SL, Gill J, Webb GR. The proximal origin of the hamstrings and surrounding anatomy encountered during repair. A cadaveric study. *J Bone Joint Surg Am.* 2007; 89:44-48.

21. Cox JM, Bakkum BW. Possible generators of retrotrochanteric gluteal and thigh pain: the gemelli-obturator internus complex. *J Manipulative Physiol Ther.* 2005; 28:534-538.

22. Meknas K, Christensen A, Johansen O. The internal obturator muscle may cause sciatic pain. *Pain.* 2003; 104:375-380.

23. Swan KG Jr, Wolcott M. The athletic hernia: a systematic review. *Clin Orthop Relat Res.* 2007; 455:78-87.

24. Labat JJ, Riant T, Robert R, et al. Diagnostic criteria for pudendal neuralgia by pudendal nerve entrapment (Nantes criteria). *Neurourol Urodyn.* 2008; 27:306-10.

25. Clohisy JC, Nunley RM, Otto RJ, Schoenecker PL. The frog-leg lateral radiograph accurately visualized hip cam impingement abnormalities. *Clin Orthop Relat Res.* 2007;(462):115-121.

26. Eijer H, Leunig M, Mahomed M, Ganz R. Cross-table lateral radiograph for screening of anterior femoral head-neck offset in patients with femoroacetabular impingement. *Hip Int.* 2001; 11:37-41.

27. Lequesne M de S. [False profile of the pelvis. A new radiographic incidence for the study of the hip. Its use in dysplasias and different coxopathies.] *Rev Rhum Malad Osteoarticul.* 1961; 28:643-652.

28. Lequesne MG, Laredo JD. The faux profil (oblique view) of the hip in the standing position. Contribution to the evaluation of osteoarthritis of the adult hip. *Ann Rheum Dis.*1998;57: 676-681.

29. Dunn DM. Anteversion of the neck of the femur; a method of measurement. *J Bone Joint Surg Br.* 1952; 34:181-186.

30. Clohisy JC, Carlisle JC, Beaule PE, et al. A systematic approach to the plain radiographic evaluation of the young adult hip. *J Bone Joint Surg.*2008;90(suppl 4):47-66.

31. Troelsen A, Jacobsen S, Romer L, Soballe K. Weightbearing anteroposterior pelvic radiographs are recommended in DDH assessment. *Clin Orthop Relat Res.* 2008; 466:813-819.

32. Siebenrock KA, Kalbermatten DF, Ganz R. Effect of pelvic tilt on acetabular retroversion: a study of pelves from cadavers. *Clin Orthop Relat Res.* 2003;(2407):41-8.

33. Fuchs-Winkelmann S, Peterlein CD, Tibesku CO, Weinstein SL. Comparison of pelvic radiographs in weightbearing and supine positions. *Clin Orthop Relat Res.* 2008;(466):809-812.

34. Beall DP, Martin HD, Mintz DN, et al. Anatomic and structural evaluation of the hip: a cross-sectional imaging technique combining anatomic and biomechanical evaluations. *Clin Imaging.* 2008; 32:372-381.

35. Tonnis D, Heinecke A. Acetabular and femoral anteversion: relationship with osteoarthritis of the hip. *J Bone Joint Surg Am.* 1999;81:1747-1770.

36. Pauwels F. *Biomechanics of the Normal and Diseased Hip.* New York: Springer-Verlag; 1976.

37. Wiberg G. Studies on dysplastic acetabula and congenital subluxation of the hip joint. With special reference to the complication of osteoarthritis. *Acta Chir Scand.* 1939; 83:28-38.

38. Murphy SB, Ganz R, Muller ME. The prognosis in untreated dysplasia of the hip. A study of radiographic factors that predict the outcome. *J Bone Joint Surg Am.*1995;77:985-989.

39. Delaunay S, Dussault RG, Kaplan PA, Alford BA. Radiographic measurements of dysplastic adult hips. *Skeletal Radiol.* 1997; 26:75-81.

40. Crockarell JR Jr, Trousdale RT, Guyton JL. The anterior centreedge angle. A cadaver study. *J Bone Joint Surg Br.* 2000; 82: 532-534.

41. Tonnis D. General radiography of the hip joint. In: Tonnis D, ed. *Congenital Dysplasia and Dislocation of the Hip.* Berlin-Heidelberg: Springer; 1987:100-142.

42. Conrozier T, Lequesne MG, Tron AM, et al. The effects of position on the radiographic joint space in osteoarthritis of the hip. *Osteoarthritis Cartilage.* 1997; 5:17-22.

43. Notzli HP, Wyss TF, Stoecklin CH, et al. The contour of the femoral head-neck junction as a predictor for the risk of anterior impingement. *J Bone Joint Surg Br.*2002;84:556-560.

44. Jager M, Wild A, Westhoff B, Krauspe R. Femoroacetabular impingement caused by a femoral osseous head-neck bump deformity: clinical, radiological, and experimental results. *J Orthop Sci.* 2004; 9:256-263.

45. Beck M, Kalhor M, Leunig M, Ganz R. Hip morphology influences the pattern of damage to the acetabular cartilage: femoroacetabular impingement as a cause of early osteoarthritis of the hip. *J Bone Joint Surg Br.*2005;87:1012-1018.

46. Reynolds D, Lucas J, Klaue K. Retroversion of the acetabulum. A cause of hip pain. *J Bone Joint Surg Br.* 1999; 81:281-288.

47. Tannast M, Siebenrock KA, Anderson SE. Femoroacetabular impingement: radiographic diagnosis—what the radiologist should know. *AJR Am J Roentgenol.* 2007; 188:1540-1552.

48. Petersilge CA. From the RSNA Refresher Courses. Radiological Society of North America. Chronic adult hip pain: MR arthrography of the hip. *Radiographics.* 2000;20(spec no.):S43-S52.

49. Millis MB, Murphy SB. Use of computed tomographic reconstruction in planning osteotomies of the hip. *Clin Orthop Relat Res.* 1992;(274):154-159.

50. McKibbin B. Anatomical factors in the stability of the hip joint in the newborn. *J Bone Joint Surg Br.*1970;52:148-159.

51. Keeney JA, Peelle MW, Jackson J, et al. Magnetic resonance arthrography versus arthroscopy in the evaluation of articular hip pathology. *Clin Orthop Relat Res.* 2004;(429):163-169.

52. Kim YJ, Jaramillo D, Millis MB, et al. Assessment of early osteoarthritis in hip dysplasia with delayed gadolinium-enhanced magnetic resonance imaging of cartilage. *J Bone Joint Surg Am.* 2003; 85:1987-1992.

## SUGGESTED READING

Burnett RS, Della Rocca GJ, Prather H, et al. Clinical presentation of patients with tears of the acetabular labrum. *J Bone Joint Surg Am.* 2006; 88:1448-1457.

# Procedures

# Chondral Lesions

Corey A. Wulf • Christopher M. Larson

Cartilage defects in synovial joints, in particular weight-bearing joints, remain difficult to treat. Patient factors that contribute to the difficulty in treating cartilage defects include age and desired activity levels. Techniques to restore hyaline cartilage have been successful in the laboratory setting but have not been reliably reproduced in vivo. Much of what we know with respect to treatment of cartilage defects is based on our experience with chondral lesions in the knee. Cartilage lesions in the hip are less well understood with respect to cause, incidence, natural history, treatment, and outcomes. Historically, the standard treatment for cartilage lesions in the hip has been conservative and symptomatic treatment until joint arthroplasty was indicated. Total hip arthroplasty (THA), however, is suboptimal for younger patients who wish to participate in moderate and competitive activities and is not clearly indicated for focal chondral lesions. Joint preservation remains the goal in the management of focal cartilage defects.

The recent emphasis on joint preservation techniques in the hip has provided new avenues for treatment of cartilage defects. Hip arthroscopy provides a means whereby intra-articular and cartilaginous structures of the hip may be accurately examined without the morbidity of a surgical dislocation. Arthroscopic indications are becoming clearer and the ability to treat intra-articular pathology of the hip arthroscopically has improved. Arthroscopic treatment of cartilage defects in the hip is a natural progression as our understanding of hip mechanics improves and techniques and instrumentation continue to advance.

## ANATOMY AND PATHOANATOMY

Historically, arthroscopic techniques of the hip have been limited by the unique anatomy of the hip joint. The complex three-dimensional bony structures of the proximal femur, pelvis, and acetabulum create a small window through which instruments must be passed and manipulated. This unique anatomy limits arthroscopic access to certain intra-articular zones[1] with respect to osteochondral grafting and even microfracture in some cases. Adequate visualization of the central and peripheral compartments requires arthroscopy performed with and without traction using varying degrees of capsulotomies.

The articular surfaces of the acetabulum and femoral head are covered by hyaline cartilage. A film of synovial fluid between the articular surfaces is maintained by the labrum, which acts as a seal, allowing for the distribution of contact forces. Ferguson and colleagues[2] have used a finite model and hypothesized that the labrum's sealing effect during load application maintains a pressurized layer of fluid, which prevents solid on solid, contact thus reducing wear. Loss of labral function may lead to increased cartilage degeneration or cartilage defects. The structure of hyaline cartilage can be divided into layers—superficial (tangential), middle (transitional), deep (radial), and calcified layers. The calcified layer plays an important role in chondral injuries sustained during increases in shear forces as seen in femoroacetabular impingement. As the chondral surface of the acetabulum encounters increased shear forces during impingement, the force is transmitted to the calcified layer, which is relatively weak and ultimately the site of failure. This produces the characteristic cleavage delaminations at the labrochondral junction. This shear force can also lead to a wave sign or chondral blister, and eventual deep delamination (carpet delamination) of the articular cartilage from the subchondral bone.

The causes of cartilage injuries vary. Cartilage defects may be associated with avascular necrosis (AVN), femoroacetabular impingement (FAI), dysplasia, Legg-Calve-Perthes (LCP) disease, osteochondritis dissecans, or trauma. FAI is a common cause of chondral lesions. Injuries to articular cartilage may vary in presentation from damage to the cellular matrix to osteochondral defects. Damaged cartilage may be visible, as characterized by the Outerbridge[3] classification, or appear normal on initial inspection. Probing the articular cartilage will occasionally reveal softening or deep delamination that is not evident on initial inspection.

Cartilage lesions may be found on the femur, acetabulum, or both. Femoral lesions appear to be less common than acetabular lesions in patients who meet the indications for hip arthroscopy. Focal femoral chondral injuries can be iatrogenic, the result of hip dislocation or subluxation, or seen in association with AVN and Perthes (see Fig. 2-13A). For some conditions, such as FAI, the femoral surface may remain well preserved until late in the disease course. Thus, articular involvement on the femoral side is often reflective of advanced bipolar degenerative changes. Acetabular lesions can be associated with hip subluxation and dislocation, FAI, or secondary degenerative lesions as a result of femoral cartilage defects.

Chondral injuries may be found within specific locations on the femur or acetabulum according to cause. Most cartilage lesions treated in our practice arise in the setting of FAI.

Chondral injuries seen in association with FAI have locations based on the type of impingement. Anterolateral cam impingement typically results in labrochondral disruption in the anterosuperior zones (zones 2, 3, and 4) with eventual cleavage delamination of the acetabular articular cartilage in this region (Fig. 2-1). Anterior-superior pincer impingement can lead to a more linear posterior acetabular chondral lesions (zones 4, 5) described as a contrecoupe lesion. Cam, Pincer, and mixed-type pathology can result in chondral blistering of the acetabular cartilage described as the wave sign (Fig. 2-2). This wave sign can indicate a predelamination injury or a deep carpet delamination of the articular cartilage or labrochondral complex without intra-articular extension. Chondral lesions can also be seen that involve detachment of the acetabular articular cartilage away from the labrochondral junction (toward the lunate fossa; see Fig. 2-17A). Each of these patterns has specific management options. In more advanced cases, full-thickness chondral lesions with exposed subchondral bone are seen (Fig. 2-3). Our observations are similar to those reported by McCarthy and Lee.[4] They reviewed their findings of 457 hip arthroscopies and found the anterior and superior acetabulum to be the location of 73 % of the cartilage lesions. They also found that most anterior lesions were Outerbridge III or IV.

Chondral injuries associated with dysplasia predominantly involve both the anterosuperior acetabulum and femoral head.[5] Lesions involving the femoral head in the setting of dysplasia typically involve the superior weight-bearing portion of the head as opposed to involvement of the lateral, non–weight-bearing head-neck junction seen in FAI. In a series of hips that sustained lateral impact injuries, chondral lesions were located medially, with three patients demonstrat-

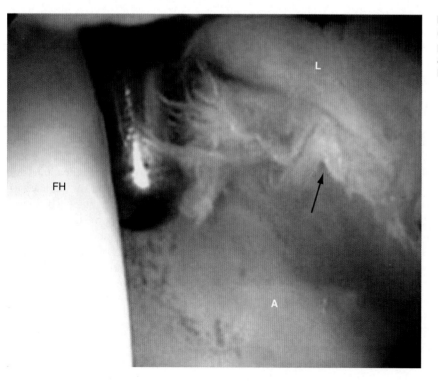

**FIGURE 2-1** Labrochondral cleavage disruption (*arrow*) in a left hip viewed through the anterior peritrochanteric portal with the shaver in the anterior portal. A, acetabulum; FH, femoral head; L, labrum.

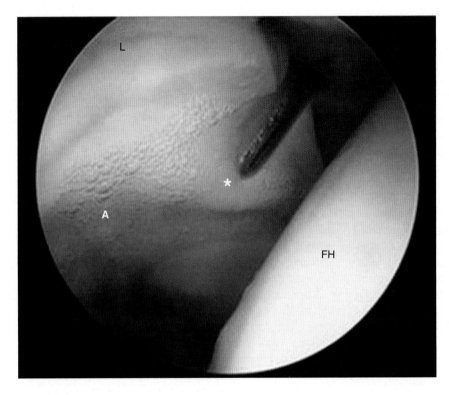

**FIGURE 2-2** Wave sign—carpet delamination—in a right hip as viewed through the anterior peritrochanteric portal, with an arthroscopic knife in the anterior portal being used as a probe to reveal the pathologic buckling or crest (*asterisks*) of the articular cartilage. A, acetabulum; FH, femoral head; L, labrum.

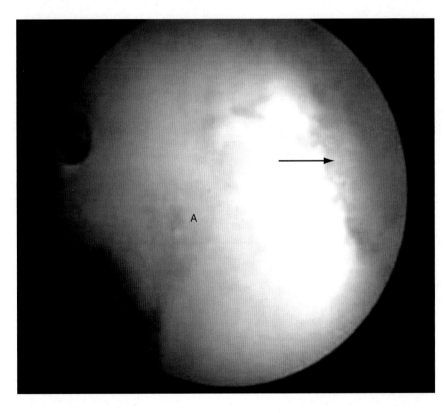

**FIGURE 2-3** Full-thickness chondral defect in the anterosuperior acetabulum (*arrow*) in a left hip viewed through the anterior peritrochanteric portal. A, acetabulum.

ing lesions on the medial weight-bearing region just superior to the cotyloid fossa and one patient with a lesion of the medial femoral head.[6] Traumatic subluxation of the hip or dislocation may also result in osseous and chondral injuries. Philippon and associates[7] reported on 14 professional athletes who were treated for traumatic dislocations of the hip, and each patient was reported to have an associated chondral lesion. Of these patients, 2 had isolated femoral head chondral defects, 6 had isolated acetabular chondral defects, and 6 had chondral defects on both surfaces. Moorman and coworkers[8] have described an MRI triad for patients who sustained traumatic hip subluxations. The triad included a lesion located at the acetabular rim, based on the direction of injury, with a posterior osteochondral and labral avulsion from the acetabulum being most common. Traumatic subluxation or dislocation may also result in AVN or osteonecrosis of the femoral head. Nontraumatic causes of AVN are also common. Regardless of the cause, AVN most commonly results in osteochondral lesions of the anterosuperior femoral head. If subchondral collapse occurs, this typically leads to further degenerative changes throughout the hip.

## HISTORY

A thorough history and physical examination are essential when evaluating patients with suspected chondral lesions. A history of traumatic injury may be noted, such as hip subluxation, dislocation, or a fall directly onto the lateral hip (Fig. 2-4). More often, there is an insidious onset of hip pain, as seen in patients with FAI (Fig. 2-5). Patients with intra-articular pathology may complain of pain in the groin or anterior or deep lateral aspect of the hip. Occasionally, symptoms are referred to the posterior-buttock region or are a combination of anterior and posterior pain, as indicated by the C sign.[9] Pain and discomfort are often exacerbated by activities such as running, cutting and pivoting in athletic endeavors, getting in

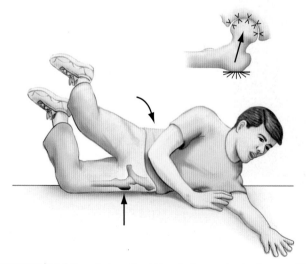

**FIGURE 2-4** A fall results in a direct blow to the greater trochanter with intact bony structure. The force generated is transferred unchecked to the hip joint. *(Courtesy of Dr. JW Thomas Byrd, Nashville.)*

and out of a car, arising from a seated position, and prolonged sitting. Patients occasionally note mechanical symptoms such as clicking, catching, or locking. In our experience clunking is more often associated with coxa saltans and not labral or chondral pathology. These complaints are indicative of intra-articular pathology and not specific to chondral injuries.

## PHYSICAL EXAMINATION

It is important to perform a complete physical examination on patients with expected chondral lesions. As noted, chondral injury and lesions are most often associated with some sort of structural abnormality (FAI, dysplasia). Evaluation and documentation of range of motion (ROM), impingement signs, and assessment of femoral anteversion in the involved and uninvolved hip are essential to determine the most appropriate course of management.

Physical examination findings associated with chondral lesions tend to be vague and nonspecific. Gait evaluation is most often normal or mildly antalgic in patients with focal chondral lesions, with the exception of acute traumatic injuries. Inspection of the patient in the supine position is helpful. In the setting of acute trauma associated with a hip effusion or hemarthrosis, the patient may hold the leg in slight flexion, external rotation, and abduction. This position places the joint capsule at maximal volume and is a more comfortable position. Palpation of the involved hip should include the following areas: groin, trochanteric and peritrochanteric regions, anterior and inferior iliac spines, buttocks, lumbar spine, pubic rami and symphysis, insertion of the rectus abdominus, external oblique, and adductor origins. Extra-articular pain often accompanies intra-articular pathology and the primary or initial source of pain should be sought. Motion may be limited by guarding in the traumatic or chronic setting because of synovitis of the hip. The Stinchfield test and supine log roll test assess hip irritability and are suggestive of an intra-articular process.[9] ROM, in particular internal rotation and flexion, may be limited in the setting of FAI. Alternatively, ROM may also be relatively increased in the setting of dysplasia or increased femoral anteversion. When performing provocative tests, it is imperative to verify whether the elicited pain is in fact the presenting complaint.

## DIAGNOSTIC IMAGING

Initial imaging evaluation includes anteroposterior pelvis, false profile, and lateral hip radiographs. The anteroposterior radiograph should have the coccyx centered over the symphysis with 0 to 3 cm between these two structures. Plain radiographs can reveal rim fractures in the setting of hip dislocation or subluxation and structural abnormalities such as FAI, dysplasia, AVN, LCP, or loose bodies. Any significant joint space narrowing should be noted as this may significantly impact the success of hip arthroscopy. In the setting of hip subluxation or dislocation, Judet views allow for better assessment of the acetabulum, specifically the acetabular rim. Various radiographic measurements are routinely performed to understand the cause of the

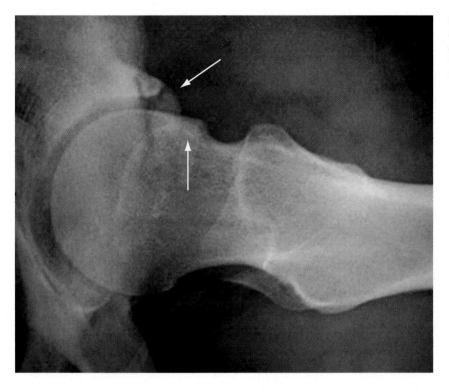

**FIGURE 2-5** Frog-leg lateral view of the left hip in a patient with combined cam (*thick white arrow*) and pincer impingement. The pincer component (*thin white arrow*) is secondary to the os acetabuli–rim fracture.

intra-articular pathology better. Our routine measurements and evaluation include the lateral center edge angle, anterior center edge angle, Tonnis angle, presence of femoral head lateralization, AP and lateral alpha angles, presence of a crossover sign, prominent ischial spines, coxa profunda or protrusio, os acetabuli or rim fractures, neck shaft angle, and Tonnis grading for degenerative changes.

Computed tomography (CT) scans are helpful for further defining fractures, loose bodies, and structural abnormalities. In the setting of an acute subluxation, a CT scan is helpful to assess for posterior or, less commonly anterior, rim fractures. A concomitant radiographically guided aspiration can also aid in decompressing a traumatic hemarthrosis when present. We frequently obtain three-dimensional reconstructions for patients with FAI (Fig. 2-6). We find that it is helpful for defining the extent of impingement and planning the rim resection and proximal femoral osteochondroplasty commonly associated with most chondral lesions.

Magnetic resonance imaging (MRI) and MR arthrography (MRA) provide better assessment of soft tissues as well as more accurate staging of AVN. Nonarthrography MRI offers the advantage of being noninvasive but with less accuracy in identifying labral and chondral pathology. When assessing labral tears, Czerny and colleagues[12] found that the sensitivity of MR arthrography was 90% and its accuracy was 91%, whereas the sensitivity of MRI was 30% and its accuracy was 36%, compared with open surgical findings. MRA, however is less sensitive for diagnosing chondral lesions in comparison to labral pathology. Keeney and associates[13] published their results comparing MRA with hip arthroscopy. With respect to articular cartilage pathology, MRA had a sensitivity of 47%, specificity of 89%, positive predictive value of 84%, negative predictive value of 59%, and accuracy of 67%. The addition of a diagnostic anesthetic injection is helpful to verify the hip joint proper as the source of pain.[33] New delayed gadolinium-enhanced magnetic resonance im-

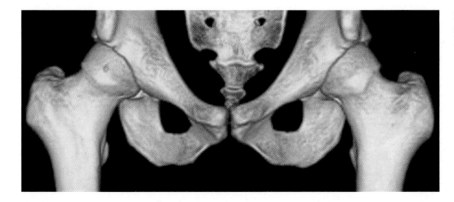

**FIGURE 2-6** Three-dimensional reconstruction CT scan of a patient with bilateral anterosuperior cam lesions of the proximal femurs.

aging of cartilage (dGEMRIC) MRI techniques may lead to improved detection of subtle chondral lesions.[15]

## INDICATIONS AND CONTRAINDICATIONS

Current treatment of cartilage lesions in the hip has evolved in recent years with the application of procedures aimed at mechanical and biologic measures to restore function and delay or prevent further degenerative changes. Indications for treatment, surgical and nonsurgical, continue to evolve as outcomes are reported. What is presented in this chapter represents indications, contraindications, and preferred treatment methods according to recent evidence-based studies and our clinical experience in a high-volume hip arthroscopy practice.

Surgery is considered for patients with suspected chondral lesions and continued pain and dysfunction, despite conservative measures and activity modification, if reasonable. Age and desired activity levels are considered when discussing treatment options. Intra-articular mechanical symptoms such as locking, catching, or clicking are indicative of loose bodies or unstable cartilage lesions. The presence of loose bodies and mechanical symptoms, which can be associated with AVN, LCP, FAI, or prior hip dislocation or subluxation, have the potential to cause third-body wear and is one of the clearest indications for surgical treatment. Patients with hip impingement can be expected to have some degree of chondral damage; they make up a significant portion of patients undergoing hip arthroscopy. Concomitant management of impingement and labral pathology, in addition to chondral lesions, should be carried out to optimize outcomes. Arthroscopy for hip dysplasia must be entertained with extreme caution because arthroscopy alone will not correct the underlying pathologic forces at work. In a patient with very mild dysplasia, arthroscopy can be considered, with every attempt made to preserve the labrum, avoid rim resection, and preserve and or repair capsulotomies during the procedure.

Contraindications to arthroscopic treatment of chondral injuries must be kept in perspective to optimize outcomes. Patients with moderate or severe osteoarthritis and a predominance of aching pain provide little opportunity for significant improvement, even in the short term. A recent study by Larson and coworkers[15] found a high rate of failure in hips with more than 50% joint space narrowing, bipolar grade 3 and 4 lesions seen on MRI scans, and a predominance of aching pain at rest. Chondral lesions greater than 2 cm in diameter also resulted in high rates of failure. Patients with significant dysplasia (center edge angle less than 20 degrees) cannot have normal joint reaction forces re-established with an arthroscopic procedure. It is critical to differentiate FAI from dysplasia because cam lesions have been reported in the presence of acetabular dysplasia.[34] The inability to restore relatively normal biomechanics can lead to failure of any cartilage restoration procedure and is therefore considered a relative contraindication to arthroscopic surgery. In addition, aggressive capsulotomies and labral débridements could lead to increased instability and failure rates in these individuals. Patients with dysplasia and superior and/or lateral subluxation on preoperative radiographs should not be considered candidates for hip arthroscopy. Finally, patients with sig-

nificant acetabular retroversion and a severely deficient posterior rim may be better served with an open procedure, such as a reverse periacetabular osteotomy, at which time any chondral defects may be addressed.

## TREATMENT

### Conservative Management

Conservative measures are appropriate initially for most patients with suspected chondral injuries. Nonsurgical management consists of physical therapy, a period of activity modification, and occasionally an intra-articular corticosteroid injection. As with any treatment decision, individual circumstances vary, and we do not apply a specific algorithm for all patients.

Physical therapy consists of core musculature strengthening and postural training. It is not uncommon for patients to have hyperlordosis of the lumbar spine and anterior pelvic tilt leading to physiologic impingement. Improved muscle balance and posture may correct their pelvic tilt and decrease their functional impingement. Increased strength and endurance about the pelvic girdle may help maintain equal distribution of joint reaction forces, therefore alleviating concentration in areas of chondral injury. For in-season athletes, it may be helpful to avoid deep hip flexion weight training such as deep squats, lunges, and clean and jerks in an attempt to finish a season prior to consideration of surgical management. Judicious use of corticosteroid injections can also be considered for these patients, but repeated injections are generally not recommended in the absence of significant degenerative changes.

Patients with degenerative arthritis are poor candidates for arthroscopy. We currently recommend therapy and symptomatic treatment, including injections and nonsteroidal anti-inflammatory drugs (NSAIDs). We will allow patients to have repeated corticosteroid injections in this setting. Kullenberg and colleagues[16] have found that pain and range of motion significantly improve at 3 and 12 weeks following an intra-articular corticosteroid injection in the setting of osteoarthritis. There is evidence in the literature to support viscosupplementation in the setting of degenerative changes in the hip,[17] but the level of evidence is low and viscosupplementation did not provide the same level of relief when compared with corticosteroids.[18]

### Surgical Management

Operative treatment of cartilage injuries in the hip represents an extension of what we have learned from treatment of cartilage injuries in other joints, in particular the knee. Microfracture is currently our primary procedure for full-thickness cartilage defects in the hip and will be the focus of this discussion. A brief review of alternative treatment options encountered in the literature will also be presented.

#### Arthroscopic Technique

**Anesthesia and Positioning.**   A general anesthetic or spinal anesthesia can be used for hip arthroscopy. Although muscle relax-

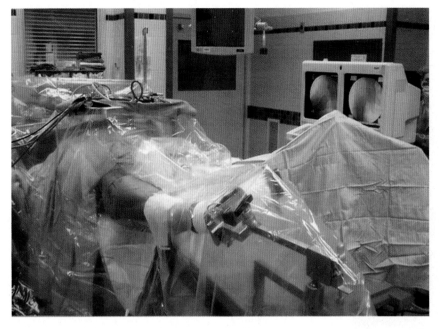

**FIGURE 2-7** Standard supine setup for a right hip arthroscopy performed on a fracture table.

ation is required for adequate distraction, paralysis is not necessary in most cases. Although hip arthroscopy can be performed in the supine or lateral position, we prefer the supine position. The patient is placed supine on a standard fracture table or standard table with the various distraction attachments available (Fig. 2-7). The involved hip is positioned in 5 to 10 degrees of flexion, neutral or slight abduction, and internal rotation. The contralateral hip is maximally abducted with external rotation. A thorough fluoroscopic evaluation of the hip is then performed. The bed is rotated, aligning the anterior superior iliac spines parallel to the floor, allowing for accurate assessment of acetabular version and rim resection if indicated. The femoral head neck junction is evaluated with the following "around the world" fluoroscopy technique. The hip is flexed to about 45 degrees with maximal internal, neutral, and external rotation. It is then extended with maximal internal, neutral, and external rotation. Finally, a cross-table lateral view with maximal internal rotation completes the evaluation of the femoral head neck junction. Distraction is then applied to verify that adequate distraction has been achieved; the distraction is then released prior to prepping and draping.

**Portals.** A standard anterior peritrochanteric portal anterior to the tip of the greater trochanter is made under fluoroscopic guidance. Saline is then flushed into the joint and backflow may reveal varying degrees of chondral debris. A spinal needle is placed in the standard posterior peritrochanteric position for outflow under direct arthroscopic visualization. We do not routinely complete a posterior peritrochanteric portal unless chondral lesions or loose bodies are located posteriorly or a posterior rim resection with or without labral refixation is required. An anterior portal is established in line with the anterior superior iliac spine and approximately one to two fingerbreadths distal to the anterior peritrochanteric portal under direct arthroscopic visualization. Making this portal distal to

the traditional portal site allows for a better angle when placing suture anchors and performing microfracture to the acetabulum. Care is taken to avoid iatrogenic damage to the labrum and articular surfaces of the hip during portal placement. Although other portals are described, a combination of these three portals allow for routine management of intra-articular hip pathology, including femoroacetabular impingement.

**Procedure.** A routine diagnostic evaluation of the central compartment is performed. A thorough evaluation is essential for defining and confirming any pathologic process, anticipated or unanticipated.[35] The anterior, superior, and posterior acetabulum, acetabular labrum, femoral head, and ligamentum teres and associated lunate fossa are carefully inspected. Chondral lesions may be obvious, as with exposed subchondral bone for full-thickness lesions or obvious displaced chondral flaps (Fig. 2-8). It is not uncommon to encounter less obvious labrochondral disruptions and it is imperative to probe the labrochondral junction thoroughly. Chondral softening or deep delamination may be noted by probing the articular cartilage; these are typically located at the anterosuperior acetabulum (Fig. 2-9). These can indicate pre-delamination injuries or deep "carpet delamination" without intraarticular extension. The size and location of the chondral injuries are recorded using the geographic zone method, as described by Ilizaliturri and associates[1] (Fig. 2-10).

The specific management technique used depends on the pattern of chondral injury and associated pathology, such as FAI. Full-thickness chondral lesions are typically addressed using the microfracture technique. Initially, any loose chondral fragments and flaps are débrided with a combination of an angled punch, ring curette, and/or shaver, taking care to leave a stable chondral edge (Fig. 2-11). It is important to verify that the surrounding chondral surface and opposing chondral surface (femur or acetabulum) have relatively healthy cartilage to ensure a contained lesion. Chondral repair techniques may

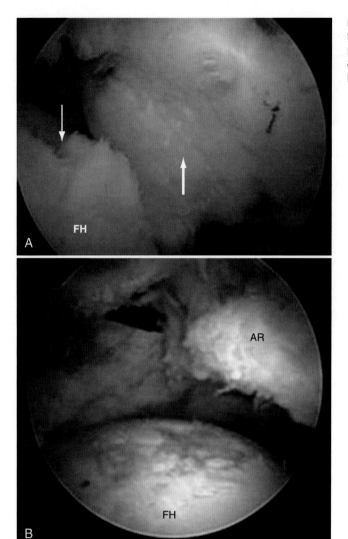

**FIGURE 2-8** Cartilage defects. **A,** Loose cartilage flap (*thick white arrow*) from the right femoral head (*black arrow*) viewed through the anterior peritrochanteric portal. **B,** Full-thickness cartilage loss of a right femoral head as viewed through the anterior peritrochanteric portal with an ablation probe in the anterior portal. AR, acetabular rim; FH, femoral head.

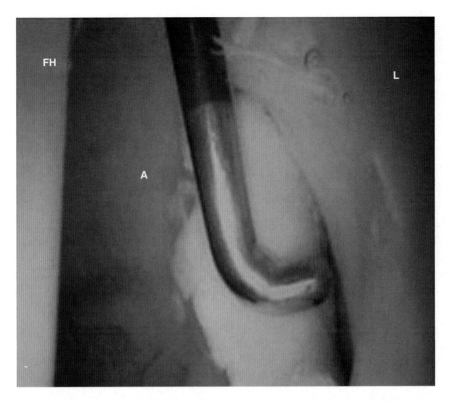

**FIGURE 2-9** Full-thickness cleavage delamination of the articular cartilage from the anterosuperior acetabulum in a left hip as viewed through the anterior peritrochanteric portal with a probe in the anterior portal. A, acetabulum; FH, femoral head; L, labrum.

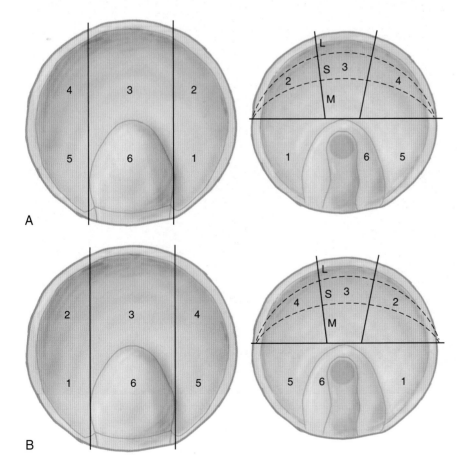

**FIGURE 2-10** Regional zone method for recording the location of intra-articular lesions. The acetabular zones are to the left. Two vertical lines are drawn using the anterior and posterior notch walls as a reference. A horizontal line is drawn at the top of the acetabular notch. These lines divide the acetabulum into six different zones. Progressive numbers are assigned to each one of the zones, starting with 1 at the anterior-inferior zone; 6 is assigned to the acetabular notch. The femoral head is to the right. Lines are positioned following the pattern of the lines used for the acetabulum. The head is presented dislocated in an open book fashion; therefore, the head is a mirror image of the acetabulum. Zone 6 contains the ligamentum teres. In the femoral head, zones 2, 4, and 5 are subdivided into three areas: medial (M), superior (S), and lateral (L). *Dashed line,* area that corresponds to the acetabular notch. **A,** Left hip zones. **B,** Right hip zones.

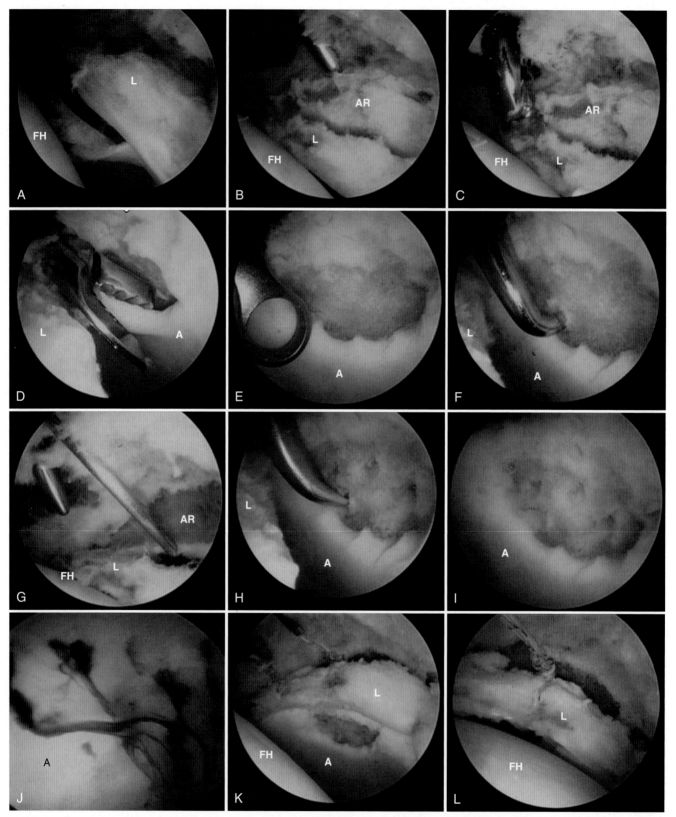

**FIGURE 2-11** Left hip in a patient with combined pincer-type and cam FAI. **A,** Typical labrochondral disruption with delamination of the articular cartilage extending medially as viewed through the anterior peritrochanteric portal. **B,** After labral takedown. **C,** Burr in the anterior portal performing a rim resection. **D,** Punch used to débride the unstable chondral flap. **E,** Ring curette used to débride the articular cartilage back to a stable rim. **F,** 90-degree microfracture awl placed through the anterior portal. **G,** Establishing a more distal and lateral accessory anterior portal with a spinal needle. **H,** 45-degree awl placed through the accessory anterior portal, **I,** Lesion after débridement and microfracture. **J,** Bleeding from the microfracture holes. **K,** After labral refixation. **L,** Traction is released, demonstrating a contained lesion with intact labrum. A, acetabulum; AR, acetabular rim; FH, femoral head; L, labrum.

not be appropriate in lesions that are not contained. Failure of containment occurs when the articular cartilage of the femoral head contacts the subchondral bone of an acetabular defect after débridement and release of traction. Similarly, failure in containment of a femoral head defect occurs when the subchondral bone of the femoral lesion contacts the articular cartilage of the acetabulum. Containment can be verified after the release of traction under direct visualization through the arthroscope or indirectly by the use of intraoperative fluoroscopy. Chondral lesions on the acetabulum are typically located at the rim and containment is readily verified with direct visualization (Fig. 2-12). Alternatively, indirect verification by observation of a well-maintained joint space on anteroposterior, frog-leg, and cross-table lateral intraoperative fluoroscopy views may indicate appropriate containment.

After removal of unstable chondral flaps, a ring curette is used to remove the calcified cartilage layer. Microfracture awls are then used to penetrate the subchondral plate, with visualization of fat droplets and or marrow elements. Microfracture begins at the periphery and ends at the center of the lesion, placing perforations 3 to 4 mm apart. Performing microfracture often requires the use of an awl through various portals. This technique provides access to the most lesions on both the acetabular and femoral head, with the exception of lesions located on the most central portion of the femoral head (medial aspect of zones 2M, 3M, 4M, and 6). Fortunately, these lie outside the major weight-bearing zones, and tend to be associated with more significant degenerative changes that would not be as appropriate for microfracture. When the microfracture is complete, the flow is stopped and subchondral bleeding is assessed to ensure an adequate depth of penetration. For hips with AVN, chondral flaps are removed to a stable edge (Fig. 2-13). Although the underlying bone is generally avascular, microfracture or deeper penetration with a drill or Kirschner wire can be performed if an appropriate angle can be achieved in an attempt to reach the deeper vascular bone.

There are other lesions with characteristic patterns of associated impingement that deserve special note. It is imperative to address any underlying femoroacetabular impingement to eliminate the cause of associated chondral lesions. This includes correction of pincer-type impingement with acetabular rim resection and cam-type impingement with femoral resection osteochondroplasty, as dictated by the nature of the impingement. Chondral treatment will likely fail if hip impingement is not corrected. For patients with pincer impingement, rim resection may eliminate or significantly decrease the size of the chondral lesion requiring treatment. Deep chondral delamination involving the labrochondral junction without intra-articular extension (carpet delamination) is another characteristic finding that can be associated with FAI (Fig. 2-14). In this situation, the labrum either requires labral resection or débridement or a careful detachment of the labrum from the articular cartilage to access the deep delamination.

We prefer to detach the labrum from the rim with a beaver blade. This is begun with the beaver blade introduced through the anterior portal and detaching the labrum to the superior extent of the lesion. The arthroscope can then be switched to the anterior portal and the labrum can be further detached superiorly and posteriorly, if necessary, with visualization obtained by inserting the arthroscope between the detached labrum and acetabulum. The beaver blade is then introduced through the anteroparatrochanteric portal between the previously detached portion of the labrum and acetabular rim (Fig. 2-15). The chondral wave, or deep delamination, is then removed with a biter and shaver, and appropriate rim resection is performed. Microfracture is then performed as described earlier and the labrum is refixed with suture anchors placed 1 cm apart (typically, three or four anchors). Labral refixation can be performed with one limb of the suture passed under and around or through the labrum. Passing the suture through the labrum creates a mattress stitch, which may better preserve the labrum-sealing function (Fig. 2-16). Microfracture can be completed after labral refixation if the labrum obstructs the view of the chondral lesion prior to refixation. Another pattern of injury involves chondral detachment–delamination away from the labrochondral junction (closer to the lunate fossa; Fig. 2-17). In this case, the articular cartilage is excised with a shaver and biter to the edge of the labrum. If pincer impingement is not present, the labrum can be débrided on the articular side if the periphery is stable or the labrum can be repaired with a similar technique as described earlier if the labrum is torn to or through the periphery. For any of these lesions, if delaminations or disruptions are partial thickness, the remaining stable cartilage is left in place and microfracture is not typically performed.

The final portion of the procedure involves an evaluation of the peripheral compartment and femoral resection osteoplasty is performed, when indicated. It should be noted that in patients with mild dysplasia, rim trimming should be avoided or minimal, and every attempt should be made to preserve the acetabular labrum. Additionally, closure of any extended capsulotomies should be considered to avoid destabilization of the hip joint. Capsular closure is performed with multiple heavy, braided absorbable sutures passed with a curved suture lasso device, tying the knot blindly on the periphery of the capsule (Fig. 2-18). The hip should be in extension and neutral rotation when tying the sutures to avoid overtightening of the capsular ligaments. Although we routinely perform closure of capsulotomies in mild or borderline dysplasia, it is unclear whether routine capsular closure in all cases has any affect on outcomes.

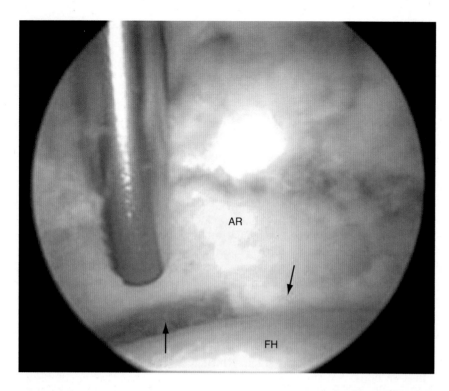

**FIGURE 2-12** Contained lesion in a right hip in a patient undergoing revision arthroscopy for residual pincer-type FAI as viewed through the anterior peritrochanteric portal, with the shaver placed in the anterior portal. The articular cartilage defect (*thick arrow*) is seen adjacent to the intact articular cartilage (*thin arrow*) of the acetabular rim (AR). The femoral head (FH) is oriented at the bottom of the image.

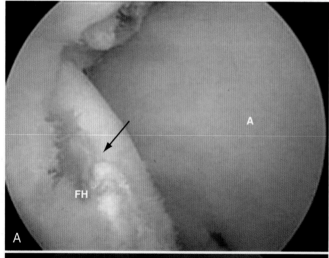

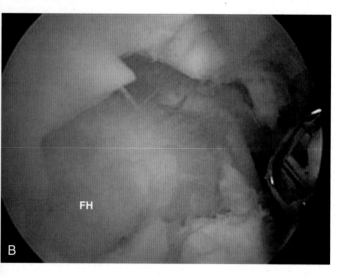

**FIGURE 2-13** Right femoral head with AVN, subchondral collapse, and full-thickness cartilage lesions viewed through the anterior peritrochanteric portal and instrumentation in the anterior portal. **A,** Full-thickness defect (*arrow*) on the anterosuperior femoral head. **B,** Further débridement with a basket punch. **C,** After removal of unstable chondral flaps. A, acetabulum; FH, femoral head.

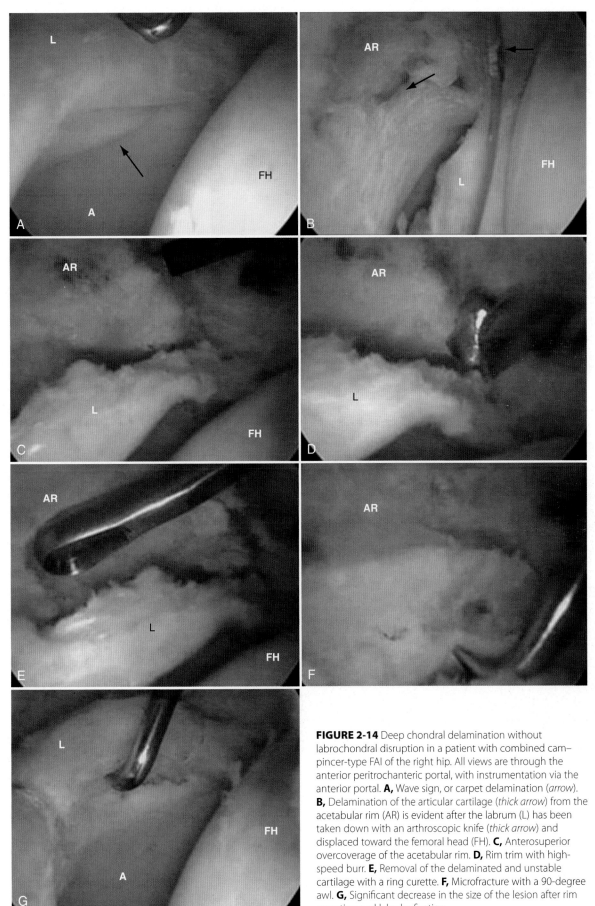

**FIGURE 2-14** Deep chondral delamination without labrochondral disruption in a patient with combined cam–pincer-type FAI of the right hip. All views are through the anterior peritrochanteric portal, with instrumentation via the anterior portal. **A,** Wave sign, or carpet delamination (*arrow*). **B,** Delamination of the articular cartilage (*thick arrow*) from the acetabular rim (AR) is evident after the labrum (L) has been taken down with an arthroscopic knife (*thick arrow*) and displaced toward the femoral head (FH). **C,** Anterosuperior overcoverage of the acetabular rim. **D,** Rim trim with high-speed burr. **E,** Removal of the delaminated and unstable cartilage with a ring curette. **F,** Microfracture with a 90-degree awl. **G,** Significant decrease in the size of the lesion after rim resection and labral refixation.

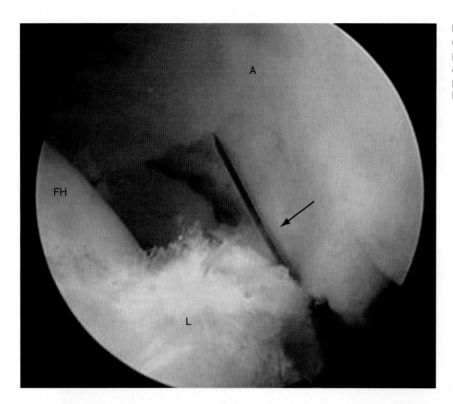

**FIGURE 2-15** Completion of the labral takedown on a left hip with the arthroscope in the anterior portal, driven between the labrum and rim. The arthroscopic knife is placed through the anterior peritrochanteric portal (*arrow*). A, acetabulum; FH, femoral head; L, labrum.

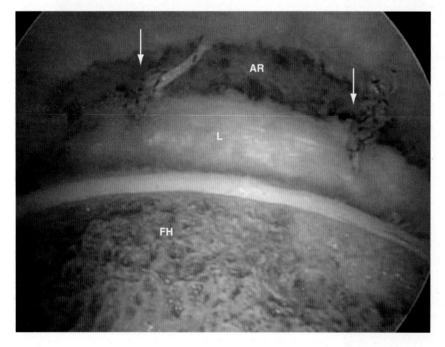

**FIGURE 2-16** Passing the suture through the labrum (*arrows*) creates a mattress stitch, which allows the labrum to sit on the edge of the acetabular rim and may restore the sealing function of the labrum better. AR, acetabular rim; FH, femoral head; L, labrum.

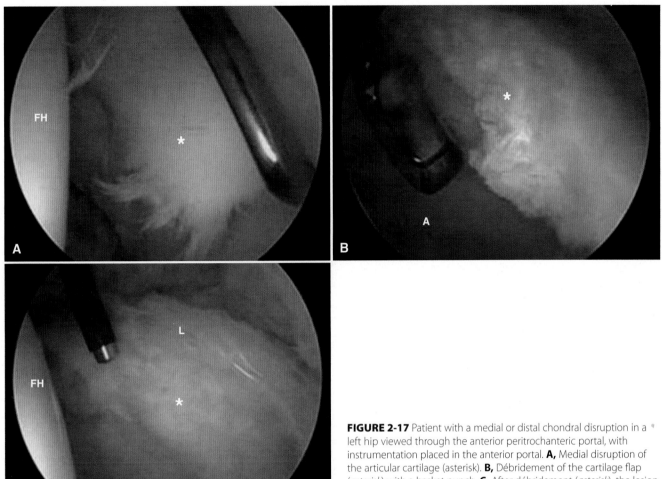

**FIGURE 2-17** Patient with a medial or distal chondral disruption in a left hip viewed through the anterior peritrochanteric portal, with instrumentation placed in the anterior portal. **A,** Medial disruption of the articular cartilage (asterisk). **B,** Débridement of the cartilage flap (*asterisk*) with a basket punch. **C,** After débridement (*asterisk*), the lesion is shown to be partial thickness and no further treatment is required. A, acetabulum; FH, femoral head; L, labrum.

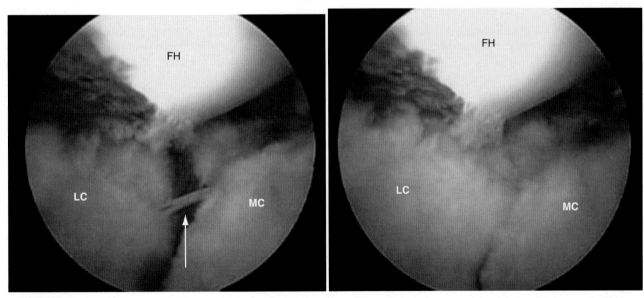

**FIGURE 2-18** Capsular closure after capsulotomy for arthroscopic treatment of FAI in the right hip viewed through the anterior portal with the femoral head (FH) oriented at the top of the images. **A,** Suture (*arrow*) is passed through the medial (MC) and lateral (LC) portions of the remaining capsule. **B,** It is then tied using an arthroscopic technique. This is typically done without visualization of the knot.

## POSTOPERATIVE PROTOCOL

### Pain Control

An intra-articular anesthetic, 0.25% bupivacaine (Marcaine) without epinephrine, is injected prior to closure of the portals when microfracture is performed. The portal sites are closed with nonabsorbable, simple sutures and a light dressing is applied. Postoperative analgesia includes oral narcotics and cryotherapy. For patients with significant pain in the recovery room, we have found that obturator nerve and lumbar plexus blocks can be of significant benefit.

### Rehabilitation

Postoperative rehabilitation is performed under the supervision of a physical therapist. Toe touch weight bearing is permitted for 6 to 8 weeks postoperatively. Early, immediate ROM is encouraged with a hip continuous passive motion machine or well-leg stationary bicycle. Gentle midrange loading is started at 4 weeks postoperatively. Core strengthening is initiated postoperatively, with care to avoid any exercises that do not comply with the weight-bearing and ROM restrictions if concomitant labral refixation is performed. At 6 to 8 weeks, progressive unrestricted strengthening is allowed, along with the addition of aerobic training and sport- specific drills, beginning at 2 to 3 months. Return to play criteria include the following: (1) full pain-free end-range loading; (2) preinjury cardiorespiratory fitness; (3) optimal sport- or activity-specific neuromuscular coordination and control; (4) trunk-hip coordinated strength = 90% of the uninvolved side; and (5) full sport- or activity-specific loading and speed with all functional drills.

## COMPLICATIONS

Complications after hip arthroscopy for chondral lesions are similar to those seen for hip arthroscopy in general. Complications include iatrogenic chondral and labral injury, nerve neuropraxias secondary to prolonged and excessive traction, broken instrumentation and, rarely, fluid extravasation. Surgeons should avoid resecting excessive acetabular rim in an attempt to minimize grade 4 lesions, because this can lead to iatrogenic hip instability. There is a significant risk for heterotopic bone formation after bony resection and psoas tendon releases in conjunction with the management of chondral lesions. Despite the potential negative effects of NSAIDs in the setting of microfracture, naproxen (500 mg twice daily) is prescribed for 2 to 3 weeks postoperatively because of the potential for heterotopic bone formation. Meticulous removal of bony debris and postoperative NSAIDs can help minimize this complication.

---

**PEARLS & PITFALLS**

**PEARLS**

1. Portals should be made distal enough to achieve an appropriate angle for placement of suture anchors or microfracture awls. Alternatively, standard portals at the level of the tip of the trochanter may be used with the addition of an accessory portal more distally to achieve proper orientation for microfracture or placement of suture anchors.
2. When angles are not appropriate with existing portals, one should not hesitate to establish additional portals verifying the appropriate angle with a spinal needle.
3. Containment should be verified to maximize outcomes after microfracture.
4. Deep delamination without intra-articular extension requires peripheral labral detachment or excision to access the labrochondral injury.

**PITFALLS**

1. Failure to address any associated impingement will likely lead to failure of chondral procedures because this is the source of associated chondral lesions in these cases.
2. Treatment of chondral injuries in the presence of significant dysplasia may lead to a higher rate of failure because the pathologic force cannot be corrected with arthroscopy.
3. Failure to gauge the degree of osteoarthritis or degenerative changes accurately may significantly affect the outcome and patient satisfaction.

---

## OUTCOMES

Current treatment of chondral lesions ranges from simple débridement to partial resurfacing with nonbiologic materials. Simple debridement provides modest relief.[19] Microfracture remains the mainstay for treatment of grade IV chondral defects, regardless of location.[20] Several authors have reported results of microfracture in the hip in small subsets of larger case series or as case reports.[21-24] Byrd and Jones[25] have reported on 21 patients with a mean follow-up of 2 years who underwent microfracture for grade IV chondral defects. Indications included a well-circumscribed grade IV articular lesion with intact subchondral bone and healthy surrounding cartilage, and the ability of the patient to participate in the 3-month structured postoperative rehabilitation protocol. The average size of the lesion was 122 mm². The mean improvement was 23.9 points (preoperative, 51.4; postoperative, 75.2). Quantitative improvement was maintained in 86% of patients. Philippon and associates[26] have reported their findings in 9 patients during revision hip arthroscopy who had undergone microfracture of acetabular lesions at the time of their index procedure. The time from index arthroscopy to revision arthroscopy ranged from 10 to 36 months. The original lesion size averaged 163 mm². Eight of 9 patients had 95% to 100% coverage of an isolated acetabular chondral lesion or acetabular lesion associated with a femoral head lesion, with a grade 1 or 2 appearance of the repair product at an average of 20 months follow-up. One patient with diffuse osteoarthritis failed, with only 25% coverage 10 months after index arthroscopy. Despite the small numbers in the current literature, the initial outcomes demonstrate promising results.

Pridie drilling has been discussed in association with open surgical approaches[27] but with no reported outcomes or arthroscopic applications. The concept is similar to that of microfracture, with introduction of pluripotent stem cells from the bone marrow that differentiate and produce fibrocartilage that fills the defect. Arthroscopic autologous chondrocyte transplantation (ACT) has not been reported in the hip with first-generation techniques and would be technically challenging. This is probably best done via an open approach. However, second- and third- generation techniques using bioabsorbable scaffolds that do not require suture stabilization may prove beneficial and applicable for arthroscopic surgery. Fontana[28] has reported non–peer-reviewed results of arthroscopic ACT versus débridement. The BioSeed-C scaffold was used for delivery of the cultured chondrocytes in a staged method. The average postoperative Harris hip score (HHS) improved in both groups. However, a greater increase was seen in the ACT group when compared with débridement alone, with scores of 86 and 65, respectively. Osteochondral autograft transplantation (OATS) and osteochondral allograft can technically be done arthroscopically for femoral chondral lesions. Medial lesions do not allow for appropriate angles of implantation but other lesions, in which an appropriate angle is achieved, can be treated with 8- to 10-mm grafts taken from the anterolateral femoral head-neck junction, with the hip out of traction. The grafts can then be implanted with or without traction, depending on the location of the lesion. This has been performed, but no peer-reviewed case reports or series have been published to date. Rittmeister and coworkers[29] have reported the results of mosaicplasty performed in five patients with osteonecrosis of the femoral head. The procedure was performed through an open approach. Four of the five had unsatisfactory results, with eventual THA at a mean of 49 months. Hart and colleagues[30] have reported their 6-month follow-up of a single patient treated with mosaicplasty. This was also done through an open approach and the patient demonstrated complete resolution of pain, full ROM, and an HHS of 100. Osteochondral allografts have also been used in the setting of AVN. Short-term results have been satisfactory,[31] but longer term results are not available in the literature. HemiCAP partial resurfacing (Arthrosurface, Franklin, Mass), has also been applied to the hip.[32]

Most of these procedures have been described through an open approach and have yet to be reported in the literature as part of an arthroscopic approach. Microfracture remains the mainstay for the primary treatment of focal chondral lesions.

## CONCLUSION

Chondral injuries in the hip remain a challenge because the surgical approaches, arthroscopic or open, have proved technically demanding. In addition, treatment options do not allow for complete restoration of normal articular cartilage. Arthroscopic removal of unstable chondral flaps and subsequent microfracture, in conjunction with the management of other associated pathology, provides promising short-term outcomes for chondral injuries in the hip. Mid- and long-term follow-up are required to determine the true efficacy and durability of these techniques. The goal of joint preservation procedures for hip disorders, which includes management of chondral lesions, is to provide symptomatic pain relief and potentially delay or prevent progressive, degenerative, hip disease.

## REFERENCES

1. IlizalitOurri Jr VM, Byrd JWT, Sampson TG, et al. A geographic zone method to describe intra-articular pathology in hip arthroscopy: cadaveric study and preliminary report. *Arthroscopy.* 2008;24:534-539.
2. Ferguson SJ, Bryant JT, Ganz R, Ito K. The acetabular labrum seal: a poroelastic finite element model. *Clin Biomech (Bristol, Avon).* 2000; 15:463-468.
3. Outerbridge R. The cause of chondromalacia patellae. *J Bone Joint Surg Br.* 1961; 43:752-754.
4. McCarthy JC, Lee JA. Arthroscopic intervention in early hip disease. *Clin Orthop Relat Res.* 2004;(429):157-162.
5. Noguchi Y, Miura H, Takasugi S, Iwamoto Y. Cartilage and labrum degeneration in the dysplastic hip generally originates in the anterosuperiorweight-bearing area: an arthroscopic observation. *Arthroscopy.* 1999; 15:496-506.
6. Byrd JWT. Lateral impact injury: a source of occult hip pathology. *Clin Sports Med.* 2001;20, 801-815.
7. Philippon MJ, Kuppersmith DA, Wolff AB, Briggs KK. Arthroscopic findings following traumatic hip dislocation in 14 professional athletes. *Arthroscopy.* 2009; 25:169-174.
8. Moorman III CT, Warren RF, Hershman EB, et al. Traumatic posterior hip subluxation in American football. *J Bone Joint Surg Am.* 2003; 85:1190-1196.
9. Byrd JWT. *Operative Hip Arthroscopy.* 2nd ed. New York: Springer; 2005.43.
10. Reider B, Martel J. Pelvis, hip and thigh. In: Reider B, Martel J, eds. *The Orthopedic Physical Examination.* Philadelphia: WB Saunders; 1999.159-199.
11. Philippon MJ, Stubbs AJ, Schenker ML, et al. Arthroscopic management of femoroacetabular impingement; osteoplasty technique and literature review. *Am J Sports Med.* 2007; 35:1571-1580.
12. Czerny C, Hofmann S, Neuhold A, et al. Lesions of the acetabular labrum: accuracy of MR imaging and MR arthrography in detection and staging. *Radiology.* 1996; 200:225-230.
13. Keeney JA, Peell MW, Jackson J, et al. Magnetic resonance arthrography versus arthroscopy in the evaluation of articular hip pathology. *Clin Orthop Relat Res.* 2004;(429):163-169.
14. Clohisy JC, Beaulé PE, O'Malley A, et al. AOA Symposium. Hip disease in the young adult: current concepts of cause and surgical treatment. *J Bone Joint Surg Am.* 2008; 90:2267-2281.

15. Larson CM, Giveans MR, Taylor M. Effect of osteoarthritis on outcomes after management of femoroacetabular impingement. Paper presented at: American Orthopaedic Society for Sports Medicine Specialty Day; Las Vegas; February 2009.

16. Kullenburg B, Runesson R, Tuvhag R, et al. Intra-articular corticosteroid injection: pain relief in osteoarthritis of the hip? *J Rheumatol.* 2004; 31:2265-2268.

17. van den Bekerom MPJ, Lamme B, Sermon A, Mulier M. What is the evidence for viscosupplementation in the treatment of patients with hip osteoarthritis? Systematic review of the literature. *Arch Orthop Trauma Surg.* 2008; 128:815-823.

18. Qvistgaard E, Christensen R, Torp-Pedersen S, Bliddal H. Intra-articular treatment of hip osteoarthritis: a randomized trial of hyaluronic acid, corticosteroid, and isotonic saline. *Osteoarthritis Cartilage.* 2006; 14:163-170.

19. Byrd JWT, Jones KS. Prospective analysis of hip arthroscopy with 2-year follow-up. *Arthroscopy.* 2000; 16:578-587.

20. Steadman JR, Briggs KK, Rodrigo JJ, et al. Outcomes of microfracture for traumatic chondral defects of the knee: average 11-year follow-up. *Arthroscopy.* 2003; 9:477-484.

21. Kelly BT, Williams RJ 3rd, Philippon MJ. Hip arthroscopy: current indications, treatment options, and management issues. *Am J Sports Med.* 2003; 31:1020-1037.

22. Hardy P, Hinojosa JF, Coudane H, et al. Osteochondritis dissecans of the acetabulum. Apropos of a case. *Rev Chir Orthop Reparatrice Appar Mot.* 1992; 78:134-137.

23. Roy DR. Arthroscopic findings of the hip in new onset hip pain in adolescents with previous Legg-Calve-Perthes disease. *J Pediatr Orthop B.* 2005; 14:151-155.

24. McCarthy J, Barsoum W, Puri L, et al. The role of hip arthroscopy in the elite athlete. *Clin Orthop Relat Res.* 2003;(406):71-74.

25. Byrd JWT, Jones KS. Microfracture for grade IV chondral lesions of the hip (SS-89). *Arthroscopy.* 2004; 20(suppl 1):e41.

26. Philippon MJ, Schenker ML, Briggs KK, Maxwell RB. Can microfracture produce repair tissue in acetabular chondral defects? *Arthroscopy.* 2008; 24:46-50.

27. Beck M, Leunig M, Parvizi J, et al. Anterior femoroacetabular impingement. Part II. Midterm results of surgical treatment. *Clin Orthop Relat Res.* 2004;(418):67-73.

28. Fontana A. Arthroscopic approach in hip defects. In: Zanasi S, Brittberg M, Marcacci M, eds. *Basic Science, Clinical Repair and Reconstruction of Articular Cartilage Defects: Current Status and Prospects.* Bologna, Italy: Timeo Editore; 2006.419-422.

29. Rittmeister M, Hochmuth K, Kriener S, Richolt J. Five-year results following autogenous osteochondral transplantation to the femoral head. *Orthopade.* 2005; 34:320-326.

30. Hart R, Janecek M, Visna P, et al. Mosaicplasty for the treatment of femoral head defect after incorrect resorbable screw insertion. *Arthroscopy.* 2003; 19:e1-e5.

31. Meyers MH, Jones RE, Bucholz RW, Wenger DR. Fresh autogenous grafts and osteochondral allografts for the treatment of segmental collapse in osteonecrosis of the hip. *Clin Orthop Relat Res.* 1983;(174):107-112.

32. Jager M, Begg MJW, Krauspe R. Partial hemi-resurfacing of the hip joint—a new approach to treat local osteochondral defects? *Biomed Tech.* 2006; 51:371-376.

33. Byrd JWT, Jones KS. Diagnostic accuracy of clinical assessment, magnetic resonance imaging, magnetic resonance arthrography, intra-articular injection in hip arthroscopy patients. *Am J Sports Med.* 2004; 32:1668-1674.

34. Ganz R, Leunig M. Morphological variations of residual hip dysplasia in the adult. *Hip Int.* 2007;17;S22-S28.

35. Bond JL, Knutson ZA, Ebert A, Guanche CA. The 23-point arthroscopic examination of the hip: basic setup, portal placement, and surgical technique. *Arthroscopy.* 2009; 25:416-429.

# Labral Pathology

Ivan H. Wong ● Carlos A. Guanche

Our understanding of labral pathology as a cause of hip pain is evolving. The exact prevalence of acetabular labral tears in the general population is unknown. Injuries to the acetabular labrum are the most consistent pathologic findings identified at the time of hip arthroscopy. In the review of their last 300 cases by Kelly and colleagues,[1] labral tears were present in 90%. Labral tears are most frequently anterior and often are associated with sudden twisting or pivoting motions.

Current surgical options, as well as the indication for surgery, are being developed. The ideal indication for labral repair would be a labral tear from a recent traumatic injury. The common presentation, however, has no inciting event, and is caused by chronic repetitive injuries that led to an attritional tear. Therefore, it is important to understand that treatment of the underlying pathology is as important as treating the labral tear, or the long-term results will be poor.

## ANATOMY AND PATHOANATOMY

The hip labrum is a fibrocartilaginous structure that surrounds the rim of the acetabulum in an almost circumferential manner. It is contiguous with the transverse acetabular ligament across the acetabular notch. The labrum is widest in the anterior half, thickest in the superior half, and merges with the articular hyaline cartilage of the acetabulum through a transition zone of 1 to 2 mm.[2] The labrum is firmly attached to the rim of the acetabulum. Its junction with the osseous margin is irregular, and there may be extension of bone into the substance of the labrum. A group of three or four vessels is located in the substance of the labrum on the capsular side of this bony extension from the acetabulum and penetrates into the peripheral third of the labrum. The labrum is sepa-

rated from the hip capsule by a narrow synovium-lined recess.[3] Extrapolating from our understanding of the healing capacity of the meniscus, repair strategies should be considered for tears involving only the peripheral labrum.

## Function

We are only beginning to understand the function of the labrum. The bony congruity of the hip joint allows for primary stability. The labrum functions as a secondary stabilizer by extending the acetabular congruity and helping maintain the negative intra-articular pressure within the joint. This has been confirmed through a poroelastic finite model that showed the labrum helps provide structural resistance to lateral motion of the femoral head within the acetabulum.[4] Furthermore, it has been demonstrated that the labrum decreases the contact pressures within the hip, probably as a result of its effect on maintaining the articular fluid in contact with the weight-bearing cartilage.[5]

## Causes of Labral Tearing

There are many theories on the mechanism of labral tearing, suggesting that the cause is multifactorial. Kelly and associates[1] have identified at least five causes of labral tears: (1) trauma, (2) femoroacetabular impingement (FAI), (3) capsular laxity and hip hypermobility, (4) dysplasia, and (5) degeneration.

Injury to the labrum could occur with traction, which would cause a tear resulting from excessive or repetitive external rotation of the femoral head on the anterior labrum.[6] Compression forces may also tear the labrum through excessive and repetitive flexion and/or internal rotation of the hip.

This process could be accelerated with FAI (see Chapter 4). Atraumatic instability has also been attributed to a deficient labrum associated with redundant capsular or ligamentous tissue that allows for more strain, and may transiently cause an incongruent joint. Deformities of the femoral head or acetabulum (e.g., slipped capital femoral epiphysis lesions, Legg-Calvé-Perthes disease, developmental dysplasia of the hip) have been discussed as a cause of labral tearing from incongruities between the femur and acetabulum.[7]

In the setting of a normal labrum, supraphysiologic loads would be required to produce a labral tear. Conversely, in the setting of an abnormal labrum, tearing could occur at physiologic loads. Sports that require repeated hip rotation, such as football, golf, gymnastics, soccer, ballet, and baseball, are susceptible to overuse injuries to the labrum and capsuloligamentous complex.[8]

Regardless of the mechanism, most labral tears encountered at the time of arthroscopy occur in the anterior quadrant. In a series by Fitzgerald,[9] 45 of 49 labral injuries were documented in the anterior marginal attachment of the acetabulum. These findings were supported by another study, which reported that 96% of labral tears encountered in a series of 436 consecutive hip arthroscopies occur in the anterior quadrant.[10]

The data from cadavers show that labral lesions are extremely common, present in 93% of specimens. Because the labrum is thought to be a stabilizing structure in the hip, labral lesions might contribute to the development of osteoarthritis in numerous ways. Injury or degeneration of the labrum may result in instability of the femoral head in the acetabulum, resulting in cartilage damage adjacent to the damaged labrum. This instability also might be more widespread, resulting in cartilage damage in the weight-bearing region of the acetabulum.[6] Finally, the lack of a seal may affect cartilage density as a result of fluid loss from the central articular compartment.[4]

## HISTORY AND PHYSICAL EXAMINATION

The clinical presentation of patients with a tear of the labrum is variable and, as a result, the diagnosis is often missed initially. Burnett and coworkers[11] have reported on a series of 66 patients in whom the diagnosis of a labral tear had been made by arthroscopy. In this series, the mean time from onset of symptoms to diagnosis was 21 months. An average of 3.3 health care providers had seen each patient prior to their being diagnosed. Groin pain was the most common complaint (92%), with the onset of symptoms most often insidious. The most common examination finding was a positive impingement sign, which occurred in 95% of patients in this series.

Most patients who present with labral injury report activity-related groin pain in the affected hip. A few patients also report gluteal or trochanteric pain, secondary to aberrant gait mechanics. In some patients, the gluteal pain may be a sign of posterior labral injury. Although most patients do not specifically report loss of hip range of motion (ROM), this finding is almost universally seen. Hips with structural abnormalities, such as acetabular retroversion, coxa profunda, or pistol grip deformities, may have decreased ROM from anatomic limitations, but may also

be limited by pain. Patients with pathologic hip conditions also commonly develop late capsulitis, synovitis, and/or trochanteric bursitis. Differential diagnosis of the classic mechanical symptoms (painful catching or clicking) of labral tears includes a snapping iliotibial tendon or hypermobile psoas tendon.[1] Many other conditions can produce symptoms around the hip. The differential diagnosis should include an array of disorders such as sacroiliitis, degenerative disk disease, abductor muscle problems, osteonecrosis, psoas tendinitis, pubic rami fractures, and stress fractures of the proximal femur. More chronic problems are usually associated with trochanteric bursitis.[12]

The physical examination for labral injuries is similar to examining for FAI. Clinical examination of the affected hip should begin with evaluation of the patient's gait and foot progression angle and measurement of leg length. The antalgic gait pattern should be differentiated from the Trendelenburg gait, seen in patients with hip dysplasia who have weak abductors. Patients with deformities secondary to a slipped capital femoral epiphysis (SCFE) may ambulate with an externally rotated extremity and open foot progression angle, more than 10 degrees. Leg lengths should be measured by using blocks in the standing position or by taking true leg length measurements from the anterior-superior iliac spine to the distal aspect of the medial malleolus. Hip pathology may be detected on inspection of the lower extremity rotation with the legs at rest. Typically, both feet rest symmetrically at approximately 10 to 30 degrees of external rotation. Asymmetrical external rotation of the legs may indicate acetabular retroversion, femoral retrotorsion, or femoral head-neck abnormalities. The hip is then carried through a ROM. One hand should be kept over the spinous process during flexion to allow immediate detection of pelvic flexion once the proximal femur contacts the acetabulum. Rotation is then measured with the hip flexed at 90 degrees. The patient with retroversion and FAI has limited flexion and/or internal rotation.

In addition to functionally limiting symptoms, reproducible physical findings, and mechanical symptoms, restricted ROM from pain or a perceived mechanical block is a further indication of an intra-articular cause. Findings on physical examination can include a positive McCarthy sign—with both hips fully flexed, the patient's pain is reproduced by extending the affected leg, first in external rotation and then in internal rotation. Also common is inguinal pain with flexion, adduction, and internal rotation of the hip, as well as anterior inguinal pain with ipsilateral resisted straight leg raising.[13] The pain, which may be of sudden onset or associated with a traumatic event such as a fall or twisting injury, is generally exacerbated with activity and does not respond to conservative treatment including ice, rest, nonsteroidal anti-inflammatory drugs (NSAIDs), and physical therapy. Conservative treatment may be successful for muscle strains but not for acetabular labral tears.

The impingement test was first described for patients with femoroacetabular impingement, but is equally useful for labral injuries. With the hip at 90 degrees of flexion, maximum internal rotation and adduction is performed. Contact between the anterosuperior acetabular rim and femoral neck elicits pain (Fig. 3-1). The hip can also be tested at varying degrees of flex-

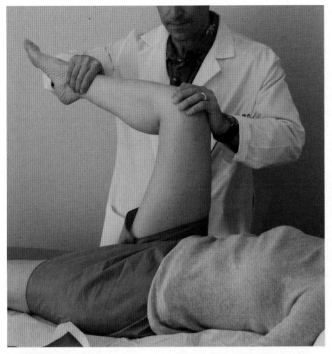

**FIGURE 3-1** Impingement maneuver. With flexion, adduction, and internal rotation, the patient's symptoms can be reproduced.

ion. Posterior labral tears can be tested with the leg externally rotated and in hyperextension.

## DIAGNOSTIC IMAGING

Weight-bearing anteroposterior (AP) pelvic and frog-leg lateral radiographs are critical in the initial assessment to evaluate the patient for arthritis and FAI, as well as subtler dysplasia.

Multiple studies have demonstrated the superior accuracy of magnetic resonance arthrography (MRA) over standard magnetic resonance imaging (MRI) for diagnosing labral tears. Intra-articular gadolinium has been shown to improve the sensitivity of diagnosing labral pathology from 25% to 92% using a small field of view.[14] Therefore, when clinical suspicion of a hip labral tear exists, MRA using a small field of view is the study of choice.

An intra-articular bupivacaine injection may be useful in situations in which the diagnosis of labral pathology is equivocal or if a tear has been diagnosed by MRA,[15] but it is uncertain whether symptoms are related to this finding. Similar to its use in diagnosing external impingement of the shoulder, if patients experience relief from their symptoms following the injection, the diagnosis of pain secondary to hip intra-articular pathology is more certain. However, intra-articular pathology could still be present without pain relief from an injection.[16]

Finally, the most sensitive test for the documentation of labral pathology is arthroscopy of the hip. With symptoms and examination findings consistent with labral pathology, and MRA fails to show a tear, it is not unreasonable to consider performing an arthroscopy for diagnostic and therapeutic reasons after a period of conservative management has

failed. Surgical intervention, however, should not be entertained until all other forms of treatment, including activity modification, physical therapy, and NSAIDs, have failed.

## CLASSIFICATION

A outcome correlated classification system of labral injuries and chondral damage has been created by McCarthy and colleagues[17] Stage 0, as compared with a normal acetabular labrum, is a contusion of the labrum with adjacent synovitis. Stage 1 is a discrete labral free margin tear with intact articular cartilage of the acetabulum and femoral head. Stage 2 is a labral tear with focal articular damage to the subjacent femoral head but with intact acetabular articular cartilage. Stage 3 is a labral tear with an adjacent focal acetabular articular cartilage lesion, with or without femoral head articular cartilage chondromalacia. Stage 4 constitutes an extensive acetabular labral tear with associated diffuse arthritic articular cartilage changes in the joint (Fig. 3-2). The labral injury involved the anterior half of the joint 95% of the time. All patients who had combined anterior and lateral labral injuries had associated degenerative arthritis in the joint.

## TREATMENT

### Nonoperative Management

Once the diagnosis of a labral tear has been made, a discussion is held with the patient regarding treatment alternatives. Conservative treatment options include avoiding activities that cause symptoms and a supervised therapy program that emphasizes hip ROM and core strengthening. Although it is unlikely that the tear will heal over time, it is possible that symptoms may stabilize to the point where the patient no longer experiences problems. If conservative management is elected, the patient should understand the need to avoid activities that produce symptoms and the possibility that the tear may progress and potentially predispose to arthritic changes in the affected hip. To our knowledge, there are no published series detailing the results of physical therapy for the treatment of symptomatic hip labral tears.

### Surgical Management

#### Arthroscopic Technique

The decision to proceed with operative intervention should be heavily weighted on refractory pain and mechanical symptoms. Most labral tears are treated with débridement. However, some tears are amenable to arthroscopic repair. As noted, the blood supply to the labrum enters from the adjacent joint capsule. Vascularity was detected in the peripheral third of the labrum whereas the inner two thirds of the labrum were avascular. Thus, peripheral tears have healing potential and repairs should be considered if this is observed at the time of surgery. However, McCarthy and colleagues[6] have reported on 436 consecutive hip arthroscopies, including 261 labral tears, and all the tears were located at the relatively avascular articular junction.

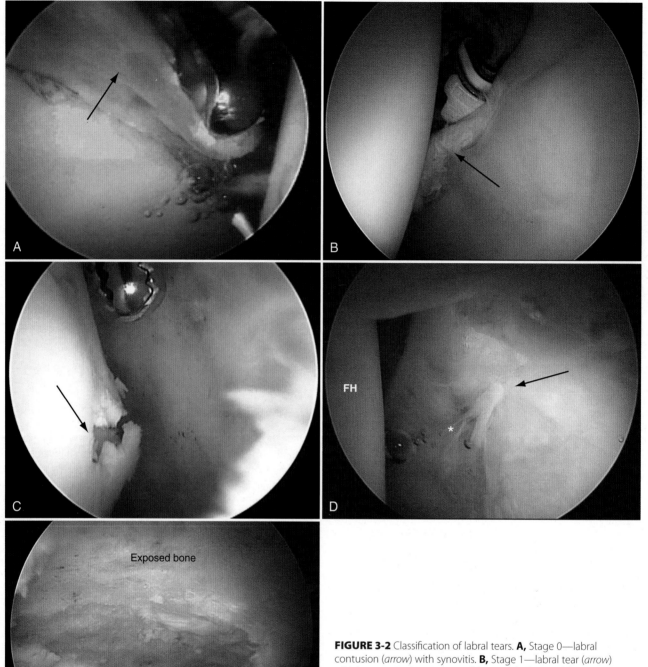

**FIGURE 3-2** Classification of labral tears. **A,** Stage 0—labral contusion (*arrow*) with synovitis. **B,** Stage 1—labral tear (*arrow*) with intact articular cartilage of the acetabulum and femoral head. **C,** Stage 2—labral tear with focal articular damage (*arrow*) to the subjacent femoral head but with intact acetabular cartilage. **D,** Stage 3—labral tear (*arrow*) with an adjacent focal acetabular cartilage lesion, with or without femoral head (FH) articular cartilage damage. **E,** Stage 4—extensive acetabular labral tear, with associated diffuse arthritic articular cartilage changes in the joint. The *arrow* delineates transition to normal cartilage.

**Arthroscopic Labral Débridement.**   It is our preference to use a general anesthetic supplemented with a lumbar plexus block for post-perative analgesia and relaxation.[18] The procedure can be performed in the supine or lateral position and should use both a 30- and 70-degree arthroscope for a thorough assessment of the labrum and any associated pathology. Modified arthroscopic flexible instruments, extended shavers, and hip-specific instrumentation should be available to improve access to all areas of the joint.

A diagnostic arthroscopic examination of the central compartment can be done systematically to evaluate not only the labrum from anterior to posterior, but also to locate possible cartilage lesions on the acetabular and femoral sides. As with the classification, the typical cartilage lesions are adjacent to injured labrum. In addition, the integrity of the ligamentum teres should be assessed. This area can be a source of pain as a result of impingement of the soft tissues between the femoral head and acetabulum. Any loose bodies should be noted and their source identified. Finally, an assessment should be made of any obvious capsular redundancy or laxity.

Many patients will have a significant synovitis associated with the labral tearing and an effort should be made to resect some of the inflamed tissue, not only for visualization of the joint but also to decrease the associated pain. It is our preference to use a radiofrequency (RF) probe to decrease the potential for bleeding and subsequent compromise of the surgical field.

The goal of the surgical procedure should be to preserve as much tissue as is technically feasible while resecting the degenerative or damaged material. This is important to maintain the labrum's role as a secondary joint stabilizer and minimize the potential for arthrosis. Fraying from the labral tears should be débrided with the use of motorized shavers or RF probes. Placing absorbable suture through the defect and tying the suture through the capsule can stabilize intrasubstance labral tears. It is important to delineate the areas of abnormal tissue identified on radiographs (in the form of perilabral calcifications) and on MRA and MRI scans (abnormal signal intensity) to address the labral pathology thoroughly. Occasionally, perilabral calcifications can be in the formative stage; these should be sought out and decompressed (Fig. 3-3).

Adjacent cartilage damage should be sought and thoroughly assessed. Superficial lesions can be gently débrided with mechanical shavers and perhaps stabilized with the use of RF probes. Grade IV Outerbridge lesions may be managed with a thorough débridement down to a bleeding bed and preparation with microfracture awls (Fig. 3-4).

**Arthroscopic Labral Repair.**   The decision to perform a labral repair is still a process in its infancy. The current indications are symptomatic tears that have obvious vascularity within their substance or are reparable to the acetabular bony wall or adjacent capsule. In general, a tear less than 1cm in length does not require repair because there are minimal associated instability and mechanical symptomatology. Expert arthroscopic skills and appropriate instrumentation are also required to perform this repair. It can be performed in the supine or lateral position under general anesthesia, often supplemented with a lumbar plexus block (see earlier).

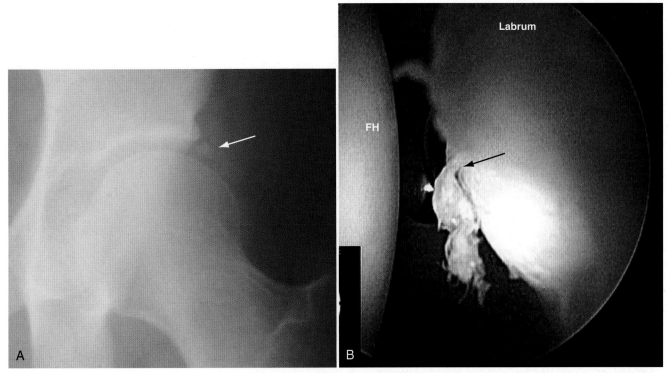

**FIGURE 3-3** Perilabral calcification. **A,** AP radiograph depicting perilabral calcification (*arrow*). **B,** Arthroscopic view of left hip from the anterolateral portal showing decompression of calcified material (*arrow*). FH, femoral head.

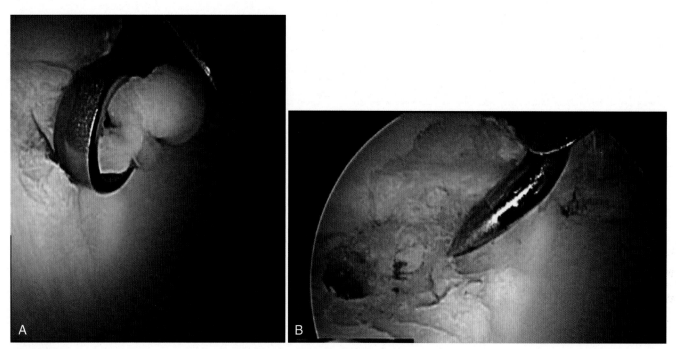

**FIGURE 3-4** Microfracture steps in a right hip viewed from the anterolateral portal. **A,** Initial lesion with curette in place working from the anterior portal. **B,** Creation of bleeding bed with awl in place.

Best results can be expected with operations with the correct indications, as follows:

■ Mechanical symptoms with rotational activities
■ Unremitting groin pain with weight-bearing activities
■ Concomitant FAI with healthy reparable tissue
■ Traumatic dislocation or subluxation with ongoing mechanical symptoms
■ Subluxation episodes in high-performance athletes

■ Tissue with obvious vascularity in proper (capsular) anatomic zone
■ Tears larger than 1 cm

The arthroscopic technique uses routine anterior and anterolateral portals and an accessory midanterior portal that is halfway between the two portals and 5 cm distal (Fig. 3-5). This accessory portal allows for a more appropriate angle for suture anchor placement. However, caution should

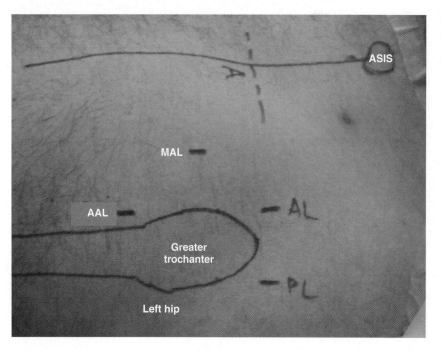

**FIGURE 3-5** Midanterolateral portal (MAL). The portal is created approximately halfway between the standard anterior portal (A) and the anterolateral portal (AL), creating an equilateral triangle between the points. AAL, accessory anterolateral portal; ASIS, anterior superior iliac spine; PL, posterolateral portal.

be taken in creating this portal because excessively distal placement places the ascending lateral circumflex artery at risk, with the possibility of bleeding and compromise of the surgical field.[19]

As with labral débridement, the procedure includes a diagnostic arthroscopy, with treatment of any associated pathology. Any degenerative tissue is débrided, and the labrum is elevated from the bone. The bony bed is prepared by decorticating with a curette or shaver to stimulate healing (Fig. 3-6).

One important consideration is to develop adequate access to the joint. Unlike the shoulder, the hip capsule is significantly thicker and less forgiving with respect to maneuverability within the joint. Therefore, a generous capsulotomy should be considered in many cases so that instruments can be moved within the joint and to limit the amount of iatrogenic damage to the articular cartilage. The capsulotomy can be performed with an arthroscopic knife or RF probe (Fig. 3-7). In addition, the use of slotted cannulas can make delivery of curved instruments significantly easier (Fig. 3-8). These devices are available in a variety of lengths and circumferences to allow their use in the hip.

Similar to arthroscopic labral repair in the shoulder, suture anchors are effective to reattach labrum to bone. The position of the anchor is critical in re-establishing the normal anatomy of the labrum. It should be placed on the ac-

etabular rim, with care to avoid penetrating into the articular cartilage. In contrast to the shoulder, the acetabular cavity is concave. This makes the requisite angle of the anchor insertion significantly more acute. Avoiding chondral injury, both to the head (delivery of the anchor) and with respect to acetabular penetration, is important, because it can become a factor in joint degeneration. Both endoscopic and fluoroscopic visualization are essential (Fig. 3-9). There are many options for suture anchors, some requiring traditional arthroscopic knot tying; knotless type anchors have recently been developed (Fig. 3-10).

Once the anchor is placed, a suture-passing device is used to penetrate the labrum and standard knot-tying techniques may be used. Most available instruments have been adapted from those used in shoulder arthroscopy.

With a tear in the labrocapsular junction, the repair can be performed, attaching the labrum to the adjacent capsular tissue. Intrasubstance tears may be addressed in a similar manner. The cleavage plane in the labrum should be defined and débrided of nonviable tissue. A suture shuttle device can be used to deliver a looped monofilament suture between the junction of the articular cartilage and the fibrocartilage labrum. A suture penetrator is used through the capsule to grasp the loop of monofilament. The looped shuttle is used to shuttle a monofilament suture around the labral tear and through the capsule. The suture is then tied in an extra-articular position.

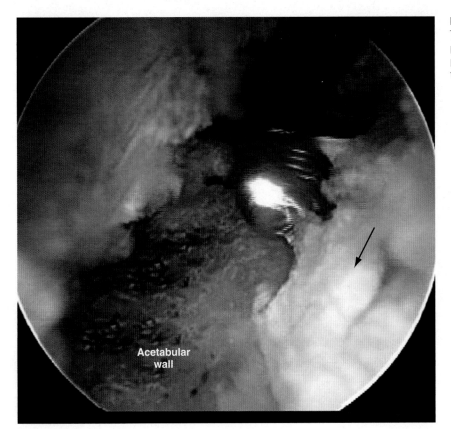

**FIGURE 3-6** Bony bed preparation for labral repair. This right hip is viewed from the anterolateral portal, and the burr is being used from the anterior portal. The *arrow* indicates the retracted labral tissue.

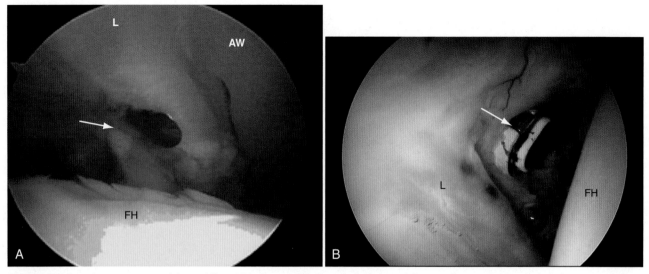

**FIGURE 3-7** Capsulotomy to expand the mobility within the portal **A,** Use of a knife (*arrow*) for capsulotomy. **B,** Use of a radiofrequency probe (*arrow*). AW, acetabular wall; fh, femoral head l, labrum.

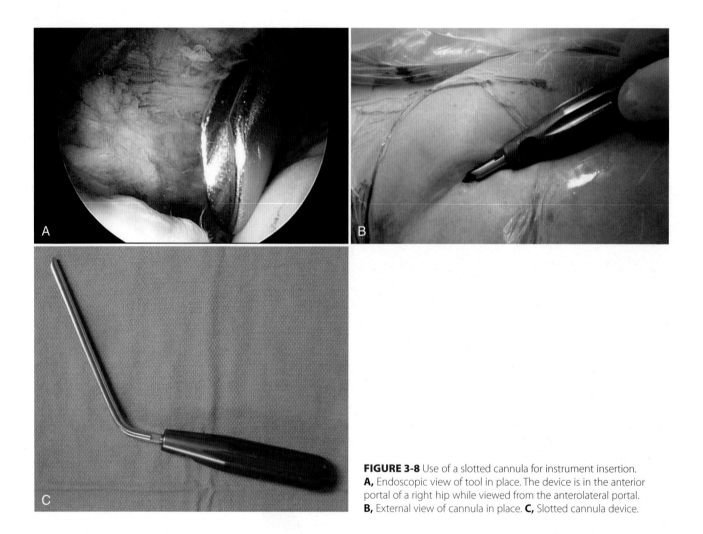

**FIGURE 3-8** Use of a slotted cannula for instrument insertion. **A,** Endoscopic view of tool in place. The device is in the anterior portal of a right hip while viewed from the anterolateral portal. **B,** External view of cannula in place. **C,** Slotted cannula device.

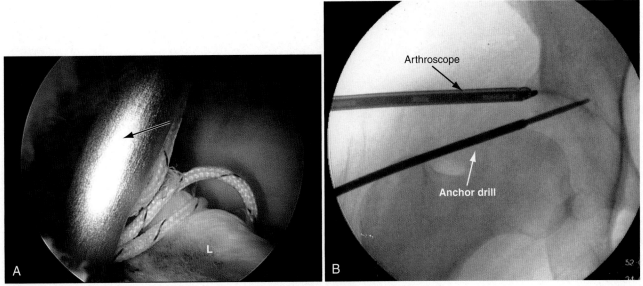

**FIGURE 3-9** Fluoroscopic and endoscopic visualization of anchor insertion point. **A,** Endoscopic view of anchor cannula (*arrow*) in place from the anterior portal while viewed from the anterolateral portal in a right hip. **B,** Fluoroscopic view of insertion point. L, labral tissue with circumferential suture in place.

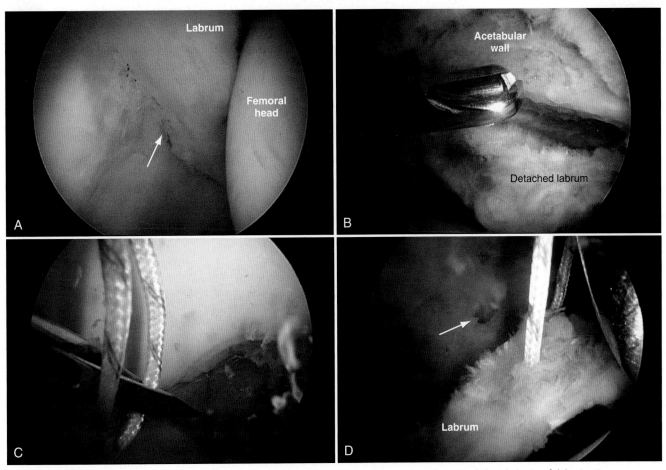

**FIGURE 3-10** Repair of labrum using a knotless technique. This is a right hip in a patient with an associated chondral area of delamination. **A,** Initial view of tear from the anterolateral portal. **B,** Prepared site viewed from the anterior portal. The burr is inserted from the anterolateral portal. **C,** Capture of the labral tissue with a penetrator device. **D,** Final suture mattress in place in robust tissue. The *arrow* is pointing to the prepared anchor insertion site.

*Continued*

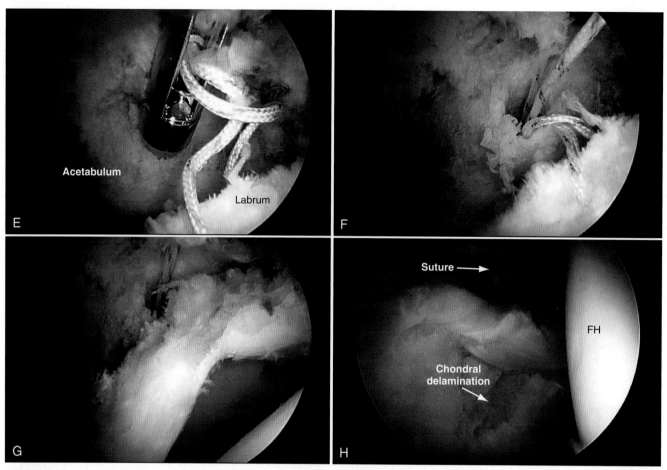

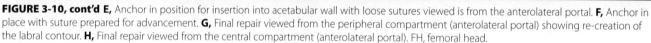

**FIGURE 3-10, cont'd E,** Anchor in position for insertion into acetabular wall with loose sutures viewed is from the anterolateral portal. **F,** Anchor in place with suture prepared for advancement. **G,** Final repair viewed from the peripheral compartment (anterolateral portal) showing re-creation of the labral contour. **H,** Final repair viewed from the central compartment (anterolateral portal). FH, femoral head.

### PEARLS & PITFALLS

- Capsulotomy (enlarge your portals for better mobility).

A beaver blade can be inserted under direct visualization in the joint. The blade can be used to enlarge the portals by opening the capsule. Any portal can be extended in this fashion to gain more mobility. This is especially important for the novice hip arthroscopist because establishment of the portals in the ideal location takes some experience. With this technique, a slightly suboptimal portal can be made ideal. Alternatively, the portal can also be enlarged with the use of an RF probe. If labral repair is undertaken, mobility within the joint is critical for appropriate position of the suture anchor and also for knot tying. The expansion of the capsulotomy is often the critical step in allowing the procedure to be completed successfully, without damaging the articular surfaces.

- Use slotted cannulas.

The use of slotted cannulas, instead of disposable plastic devices (see Fig. 3-8), makes the insertion of longer tools and curved tools significantly easier in the hip joint. For the reasons noted, the hip capsule is very restricting. The insertion of plastic cannulas is fraught with difficulties, including articular cartilage damagepon insertion. With a slotted cannula, the capsular entry point is preserved and maneuverability within the joint is enhanced compared with using a closed cannula.

- Treat the underlying pathology—look for subtle indicators of impingement.

In the broadest sense, there are two types of impingement, cam and pincer. When conducting the diagnostic arthroscopy of the central compartment, the type of labral pathology and presence or absence of chondral delamination can serve as a subtle clue of the presence of any impingement lesion.

A hypertrophic and degenerative labrum in a relatively focal area with chondral delamination directly adjacent to the labral tear is indicative of a cam lesion. If the chondral surface is intact and the labrum appears generally frayed in a more peripheral location, the situation is likely a result of pincer impingement.

- Use fluoroscopic and endoscopic visualization for anchor placement.

The liberal use of fluoroscopy while anchor insertion points are chosen allows for anchors to be placed in a safe location, with a minimal likelihood of penetrating the articular cartilage and causing iatrogenic damage. Unlike the glenoid cavity, the acetabulum is concave, making the angle of approach completely different to avoid penetration. The distortion that accompanies the use of the 70-degree arthroscope further confuses the situation and makes the use of fluoroscopy even more important.

## POSTOPERATIVE PROTOCOL

### Rehabilitation Following Débridement

Formal therapy for ROM and strengthening of the operative hip is begun 7 to 10 days following surgery. Weight bearing following an isolated arthroscopic labral débridement should be unrestricted, with the use of crutches limited to the early postoperative period only (3 to 5 days). The standard protocol includes a gradual progression from increasing the ROM to unrestricted strengthening. Strengthening is only begun once the patient attains approximately 75% of normal motion. Aggressive hip flexor strengthening should be limited until full ROM is obtained and hip mechanics are relatively normal. If patients develop abnormal mechanics to assist the recovering psoas and/or hip flexors, a significant tendinitis can develop, which is difficult to treat and slows the patient's recovery. Explosive and rotational activities should also be limited for at least 6 weeks. The return to unrestricted activity is predicated on a full painless ROM and normal strength of the pelvic, abdominal, and lower extremity musculature.

### Rehabilitation Following Labral Repair

Formal therapy for ROM and strengthening of the operative hip is also begun 7 to 10 days following surgery. Early ROM is initiated to limit the scarring in the joint associated with surgical trauma. Weight bearing following repair should be restricted to foot-flat (20% of body weight) ambulation for the first 4 weeks. The most important principle is to limit the rotational stresses that the repaired labrum experiences in the first few weeks. The range that puts the repair at risk includes flexion past 90 degrees, abduction past 25 degrees, and internal or external rotation past 25 degrees.[20] Limitations are placed on flexion past 90 degrees for 10 days, whereas abduction and abduction are limited to 25 degrees for 4 weeks. Beginning at 4 weeks, a gradual progression from increasing the ROM to unrestricted strengthening is begun. The use of stationary bicycling is encouraged and instituted in the first 10 days. Aggressive hip flexor strengthening should also be limited until full ROM is obtained and hip mechanics are relatively normal. As noted, a significant tendinitis can develop, thus slowing recovery. Explosive and rotational activities should also be limited for at least 12 weeks. The return to unrestricted activity is also predicated on a full pain-free ROM, and normal strength of the pelvic, abdominal, and lower extremity musculature. This typically occurs at approximately 4 to 6 months postoperatively.

### OUTCOMES

At a minimum of 2 years after hip arthroscopy, patient results were directly correlated with the stage of labral injury.[21] There were 11 stage 0 lesions and 1 labral lesion, with all but one of these patients having good to excellent results (91%). There were 11 patients with stage 2 labral tears, with 82% good to excellent outcomes when the tear was resected. Two patients (18%) required additional surgical intervention, including open synovectomy, capsulectomy, and release of the reflected rectus femoris tendon secondary to poor results. Patients with stage 3 labral tears did not fare nearly as well and the extent of the acetabular cartilage erosion directly affected the result, with only 17% having good to excellent results. The results of patients with stage 4 labral tears (nine hips) directly correlated with the extent of hip degenerative arthritis. If the articular cartilage involvement was diffuse on the femoral head and acetabulum, regardless of the plain radiographic appearance, the symptomatic improvement after arthroscopy was transient. At follow-up, 78% had poor results and 43% eventually had total joint arthroplasty within 2 years of arthroscopy. These results have been confirmed with the only long-term outcome study of labral débridement by Byrd and Jones.[22]

There have been numerous studies detailing the use of arthroscopy in treating lesions of the hip labrum. However, collective interpretation is confounded by the nonuniform use of outcome measures and a lack of validated outcomes for nonarthritic hip pain. Further complicating the matter is that many published series contained heterogeneous study populations in which subjects had associated hip pathology, such as arthritis, dysplasia, and FAI, in addition to labral tearing.

To date, there are no published series on the long-term outcome of arthroscopic repair of hip labral tears. Indications for which lesions constitute a reparable lesion are currently evolving. Recently, Hines and associates[25] presented outcome results on a series of 52 patients who underwent arthroscopic hip labral repair, with a mean follow-up of 9 months. Another study of 19 patients by Murphy and coworkers[23] has also recently been published. The results of these studies, as well as those documenting the outcome of labral débridement, are summarized in Table 3-1.

### COMPLICATIONS

Hip arthroscopy has been shown to be relatively safe in several studies documenting its effectiveness and the number of complications. In one large series, there was a 1.6% complication rate, with problems including transient palsy of the sciatic or femoral nerves, paresthesias secondary to lateral femoral cutaneous nerve palsy, perineal injury, and instrument breakage.[24] Although this study was not specific to the repair of the hip labrum, specific problems may be associated with this procedure. As a result of the tight confines and the multiple instruments that are inserted into the joint, the possibility of serious articular cartilage damage exists. Care should be taken while working within the joint to ensure that cartilage damage is minimal. In addition, with the insertion of suture anchors, there is a possibility of joint penetration. The liberal use of fluoroscopy to document the position of anchor insertion angles prior to committing to a specific position is critical to a successful procedure.

**TABLE 3-1**    Results of Arthroscopic Débridement and Repair of Hip Labrum Tears

| Study (Year) | Labral Treatment | No. of Patients | Mean Follow-up | Results |
|---|---|---|---|---|
| Byrd and Jones (2009)[22] | D | 50 | 10 yr | Median improvement in HHS from 52 to 81; 7 of 8 with arthritis required arthroplasty by median 53 mo |
| Hines et al (2007)[25] | R | 52 | 9 mo | 85% good to excellent |
| Murphy et al (2006)[23] | R | 19 | 6 mo | Significant improvement in HHS, SF-36, nonarthritic hip, and VAS; 67% satisfied |
| Potter et al (2005)[26] | D | 40 | 13-55 mo | 70% overall patient satisfaction |
| O'Leary et al (2001)[27] | D | 86 | 30 mo | 91% improvement with labral tears, 40% with osteonecrosis. 44% with DJD |
| Santori and Villar (2000)[28] | D | 76 | 24-61 mo | 67% overall satisfaction; mean HHS, 89.8 |
| Byrd and Jones (2000)[29] | D | 35 | 2 yr | Significant improvement in HHS; best in labral tears or loose bodies |
| Farjo et al (1999)[30] | D | 28 | 13-100 mo | 71% good to excellent without arthritis; 21% good to excellent with DJD |

*D, débridement; DJD, degenerative joint disease; HHS, Harris hip score; R, repair; SF-36, Short Form-36; VAS, visual analog score.*

## SUMMARY

The mechanical effects of the labrum appear to substantiate the need to preserve as much tissue as possible. With resection of the labrum, synovial fluid may not be contained in the weight-bearing dome of the acetabulum and is probably detrimental on a long-term basis. Therefore, the labrum should be preserved as much as possible in patients who have mechanical symptoms from labral pathology.

The available literature supports the concept that the labrum is important for stability and cartilage homeostasis. More research needs to be done to evaluate the long-term effects of labral repair or excision. It would appear that the preservation of as much relatively normal labral tissue with any surgical procedure is critical to the long-term preservation of the native hip joint.

## REFERENCES

1. Kelly BT, Weiland DE, Schenker ML, Philippon MJ. Arthroscopic labral repair in the hip: surgical technique and review of the literature. *Arthroscopy*. 2005; 21:1496-1504.
2. Seldes RM, Tan V, Hunt J, et al. Anatomy, histologic features, and vascularity of the adult acetabular labrum. *Clin Orthop Relat Res*. 2001;(382):232-240.
3. Petersilge C. Imaging of the acetabular labrum. *Magn Reson Imaging Clin North Am*. 2005; 13:641-652.
4. Ferguson SJ, Bryant JT, Ganz R, Ito K. The acetabular labrum seal: a poroelastic finite element model. *Clin Biomech (Bristol, Avon)*. 2000; 15:463-468.
5. Ferguson SJ, Bryant JT, Ganz R, Ito K. The influence of the acetabular labrum on hip joint cartilage consolidation: a poroelastic finite element model. *J Biomech*. 2000; 33:953-960.
6. McCarthy J, Noble P, Aluisio FV, et al. Anatomy, pathologic features, and treatment of acetabular labral tears. *Clin Orthop Relat Res*. 2003;(406):38-47.
7. Byrd JW, Jones KS. Hip arthroscopy in the presence of dysplasia. *Arthroscopy*. 2003; 19:1055-1060.
8. Byrd JW. Hip arthroscopy in athletes. *Instr Course Lect*. 2003; 52:701-709.
9. Fitzgerald RH. Acetabular labrum tears. Diagnosis and treatment. *Clin Orthop Relat Res*. 1995; (311):60-68.
10. McCarthy JC, Noble PC, Schuck MR, et al. The watershed labral lesion: its relationship to early arthritis of the hip. *J Arthroplasty*. 2001; 16:81-87.
11. Burnett RS, Della Rocca GJ, Prather H, et al. Clinical presentation of patients with tears of the acetabular labrum. *J Bone Joint Surg Am*. 2006; 88:1448-1457.
12. Sierra RJ, Trousdale RT, Ganz R, Leunig M. Hip disease in the young, active patient: evaluation and nonarthroplasty surgical options. *J Am Acad Orthop Surg*. 2008; 16:689-703.
13. McCarthy JC. The diagnosis and treatment of labral and chondral injuries. *Instr Course Lect*. 2004; 53:573-577.
14. Toomayan GA, Holman WR, Major NM, et al. Sensitivity of MR arthrography in the evaluation of acetabular labral tears. *AJR Am J Roentgenol*. 2006; 186:449-453.
15. Byrd JW, Jones KS. Diagnostic accuracy of clinical assessment, magnetic resonance imaging, magnetic resonance arthrography, and intra-articular injection in hip arthroscopy patients. *Am J Sports Med*. 2004; 32:1668-1674.
16. Martin RL., Irrgang JJ, Sekiya JK. The diagnostic accuracy of a clinical examination in determining intra-articular hip pain for potential hip arthroscopy candidates. *Arthroscopy*. 2008; 24:1013-1018.
17. McCarthy J, Wardell S, Mason J, et al. Injuries to the acetabular labrum: classification, outcome, and relationship to degenerative arthritis. Paper presented at: American Academy of Orthopedic Surgeons 64th Annual Meeting; February 1997; San Francisco.
18. Marino J, Russo J, Kenny M, et al. Continuous lumbar plexus block for postoperative pain control after total hip arthroplasty. A randomized controlled trial. *J Bone Joint Surg Am*. 2009; 91:29-37.
19. Robertson WJ, Kelly BT. The safe zone for hip arthroscopy: a cadaveric assessment of central, peripheral, and lateral compartment portal placement. *Arthroscopy*. 2008; 24:1019-1026.
20. Ikeda T, Awaya G, Suzuki S, et al. Torn acetabular labrum in young patients. Arthroscopic diagnosis and management. *J Bone Joint Surg Br*. 1988; 70:13-16.

21. McCarthy JC, Noble PC, Schuck MR, et al. The Otto E. Aufranc Award: the role of labral lesions to development of early degenerative hip disease. *Clin Orthop Relat Res.* 2001;(393): 25-37.

22. Byrd JW, Jones KS. Prospective analysis of hip arthroscopy with 10-year follow-up. *Arthroscopy.* 2009; 25:365-368.

23. Murphy KP, Ross AE, Javernick MA, Lehman RA Jr. Repair of the adult acetabular labrum. *Arthroscopy.* 2006; 22:567.e1-.e3.

24. Griffin DR, Villar RN. Complications of arthroscopy of the hip. *J Bone Joint Surg Br.* 1999; 81:604-606.

25. Hines SL, Philippon MJ, Kuppersmith D. Early clinical results in a group of patients undergoing hip labral repairs. Paper presented at: Annual Arthroscopy Association of North America 2007.Annual Meeting; August-September 2007; San Francisco.

26. Potter BK, Freedman BA, Andersen RC, et al. Correlation of Short Form-36 and disability status with outcomes of arthroscopic acetabular labral debridement. *Am J Sports Med.* 2005; 33:864-870.

27. O'Leary JA, Berend K, Vail TP. The relationship between diagnosis and outcome in arthroscopy of the hip. *Arthroscopy.* 2001; 17:181-188.

28. Santori N, Villar RN. Acetabular labral tears: result of arthroscopic partial limbectomy. *Arthroscopy.* 2000; 16:11-15.

29. Byrd JW, Jones KS. Prospective analysis of hip arthroscopy with 2-year follow-up. *Arthroscopy.* 2000; 16:578-587.

30. Farjo LA, Glick JM, Sampson TG. Hip arthroscopy for acetabular labral tears. *Arthroscopy.* 1999; 15:132-137.

# Cam-Type Femoroacetabular Impingement

J. W. Thomas Byrd

Surgical correction of various hip impingement problems was described even early in the last century.[1,2] In 1975, Harris and coauthors described the pistol grip deformity of the femoral head observed in association with early-onset osteoarthritis.[3] In 1998, we described arthroscopic correction of impingement caused by post-traumatic osteophytes and also reported an arthroscopic technique of cheilectomy for femoral protuberances associated with Legg-Calvé-Perthes disease.[4,5] However, it was Myers, Ganz, Lavigne and colleagues[6-8] who formulated the concept of femoroacetabular impingement, describing pincer, cam, and combined types. Subsequently, we have reported arthroscopic methods for correcting this disorder.[9-11]

We have identified a bimodal population of patients with cam-type femoroacetabular impingement (FAI).[11] One is the typical middle-aged patient (average age, 43 years, with a 1.9:1 male-to-female ratio) who presents with early-onset osteoarthritis. The second population is much younger, with an even greater male preponderance (average age, 20 years, with 3.1:1 male-to-female ratio) and most (70%) are involved in athletic activities. These are active individuals who have pushed their hip beyond its diminished physiologic limits and have sustained substantial joint breakdown at a young age.

## ANATOMY AND PATHOANATOMY

Cam-type FAI refers to the cam effect created by a nonspherical femoral head. During flexion, the prominence of the out-of-round portion rotates into the acetabulum, engaging against its surface and resulting in delamination and failure of the acetabular articular cartilage (Fig. 4-1). Early in the disease

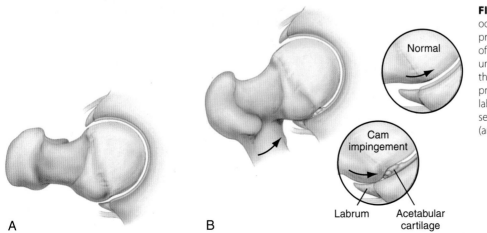

**FIGURE 4-1 A,** Cam impingement occurs with hip flexion as the bony prominence of the nonspherical portion of the femoral head (cam lesion) glides under the labrum. engaging the edge of the articular cartilage and resulting in progressive delamination. **B,** Initially, the labrum is relatively preserved, but secondary failure occurs over time (arrow).

Normal

Cam impingement

Labrum    Acetabular cartilage

A

B

process, the labrum is relatively preserved but, with time, it begins to sustain secondary damage.

Cam impingement is classically attributed to a slipped capital femoral epiphysis, resulting in a bony prominence of the anterior and anterolateral head-neck junction. However, the most common cause is the pistol grip deformity, attributed to a developmental abnormality of the capital physis during growth. The exact cause is unclear; it may represent premature asymmetrical closure of the physis; it has been postulated that this could be caused by late separation of the common proximal femoral growth plate that forms the physis of the greater trochanter and femoral head.[12]

Femoroacetabular impingement is still incompletely understood. The pathomechanics explain the observations of secondary joint pathology caused by the impingement. However, some individuals with impingement shaped hips may never become symptomatic as a result of secondary damage. Thus, it is possible to have impingement morphology without impingement pathology. The arthroscope has become invaluable in the treatment algorithm for patients with FAI. Arthroscopic observations on the secondary articular and labral damage associated with pathologic impingement dictate the need for correcting the underlying bony abnormalities.

## HISTORY AND PHYSICAL EXAMINATION

Patients with cam impingement have typical hip joint–type symptoms.[13] The onset may be gradual or associated with an acute episode, which is the culmination of altered wear developing over a protracted period of time. Patients with cam impingement usually have reduced joint motion, which can result in other secondary disorders. Athletes compensate with increased pelvic motion, often resulting in problems with athletic pubalgia.[14] More stress is placed on the lumbar spine, resulting in concomitant lumbar disease.

Pain with flexion, adduction, and internal rotation is almost uniformly present and is referred to as the impingement test (Fig. 4-2).[7] However, in our experience, this maneuver is uncomfortable for most irritable hips, regardless of the underlying cause, and thus is not specific for impingement. Laterally based cam lesions may result in painful abduction or external rotation (Fig. 4-3). Internal rotation of the flexed hip is usually diminished, but may be preserved in some patients (Fig. 4-4). Limited range of motion may be present bilaterally because the morphologic variation is often present in both hips.

## DIAGNOSTIC IMAGING

Radiographs are essential for the routine evaluation of impingement. A well-centered anteroposterior (AP) pelvis x-ray is important for assessing the acetabular indices of pincer impingement, but also allows observations on the cam lesion comparing both hips (Fig. 4-5).[15] The epicenter and shape of the cam lesion are variable. Thus, although the 40-degree Dunn view has been reported as the best image, we have found that no single lateral radiographic view is reliable for optimally assessing the cam lesion in all cases (Fig. 4-6).[16] Sometimes, the cam lesion is more

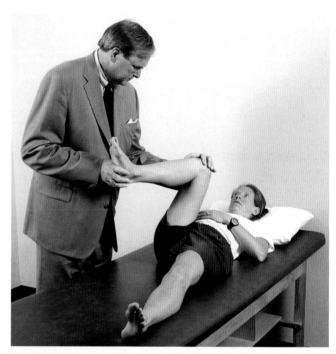

**FIGURE 4-2** The impingement test is performed by provoking pain with flexion, adduction, and internal rotation of the symptomatic hip.

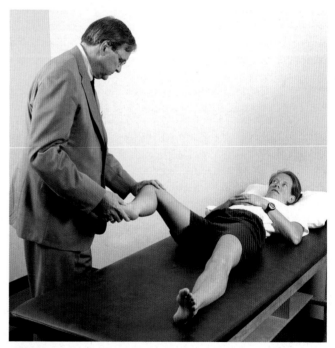

**FIGURE 4-3** Abduction and external rotation may elicit pain with laterally based cam lesions.

anteriorly based and sometimes more lateral. The characteristic feature is loss of sphericity of the femoral head. The alpha angle has been described to quantitate this observation (Fig. 4-7).[17] However, imaging will underinterpret this measurement unless it catches the maximal location of the cam lesion. Also, no studies have shown a significant correlation between the amount of correction of the alpha angle and the results of surgery, indicating that there may be other factors at play.

Magnetic resonance imaging (MRI) and gadolinium arthrography with MRI (MRA) aid in assessing secondary damage to the articular cartilage and labrum associated with cam impingement.[18] These studies are better at detecting labral pathology but reveal the severity of articular involvement less often. The alpha angle can again be recorded, but is still variable, depending on whether the cross-sectional images catch the maximal location of the cam lesion.

Computed tomography (CT) with three-dimensional reconstruction provides great clarity in evaluating the shape, size, and location of the cam lesion. This is valuable for the arthroscopic management of this condition. Exposure of the abnormal bone is simplified by knowing its exact appearance.

## INDICATIONS AND CONTRAINDICATIONS

The indication for hip arthroscopy is imaging evidence of intra-articular pathology amenable to arthroscopic intervention, or sometimes recalcitrant hip pain that remains refractory to efforts at conservative treatment. It must be kept in mind that imaging studies may often underestimate the severity of intra-articular pathology. Correction of an accompanying cam lesion has been performed, when present, especially when there was arthroscopic evidence that it was responsible for the concomitant joint pathology. This secondary joint damage is best characterized by failure of the anterolateral acetabular articular surface. The failure is most typically represented by articular delamination with the peel-back mechanism, but earlier in the disease process may be characterized by deep, closed, grade I articular blistering, referred to as the wave sign.[19]

It is our opinion that radiographic findings of impingement, in the absence of clinical findings of a joint problem, are not solely an indication for arthroscopy. Some individuals with impingement morphology may function for decades without developing secondary joint damage and symptoms. For some, it is unclear when, or if, they will develop problems warranting surgical intervention. For example, many individuals may present with symptoms in one hip when radiographic findings of impingement are present in both. Although intervention in the asymptomatic joint would not be appropriate, it is important to educate the patient about warn-

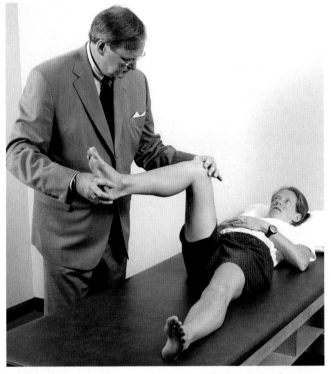

**FIGURE 4-4** Internal rotation is checked with the hip in a 90-degree flexed position.

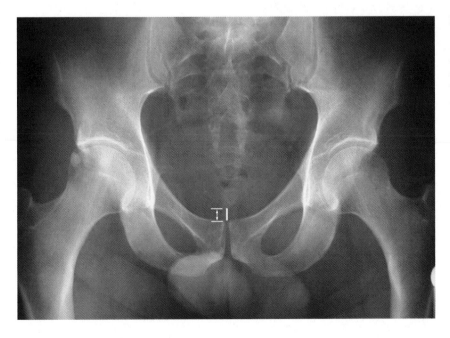

**FIGURE 4-5** A properly centered AP radiograph must be controlled for rotation and tilt. Proper rotation is confirmed by alignment of the coccyx over the symphysis pubic (*vertical line*). Proper tilt is controlled by maintaining the distance between the tip of the coccyx and the superior border of the symphysis pubis at 1 to 2 cm.

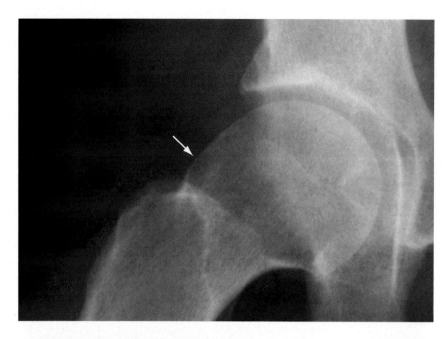

**FIGURE 4-6** The frog-leg lateral radiograph is convenient because it is simple to carry out and is reproducible. The cam lesion (*arrow*) is evident as the convex abnormality at the head-neck junction where there should normally be a concave slope of the femoral neck.

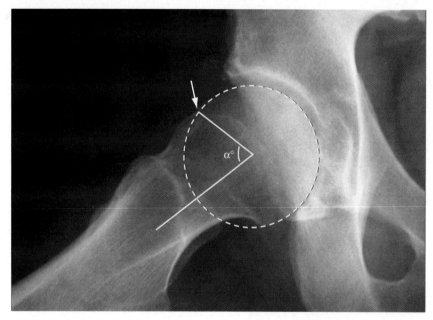

**FIGURE 4-7** The alpha angle is used to quantitate the severity of the cam lesion. A circle is placed over the femoral head. The alpha angle is formed by a line along the axis of the femoral neck (1) and a line (2) from the center of the femoral head to the point where the head diverges outside the circle (*arrow*).

ing signs of progressive joint damage. It is a clinical challenge in the decision not to intercede too early or too late. In our experience, 93% of patients undergoing arthroscopy for cam impingement demonstrate Grade III or IV articular damage, reflecting that the disease process is already substantially advanced at the time of intervention.[11]

Contraindications include advanced disease states, such as grade III Tonnis changes, and sometimes there are patients who do not have reasonable expectations of what can be accomplished with the procedure.[20] Because the success of the operation is ultimately dictated by the patient's impressions, it may be important to modulate the patient's goals. Also, in the presence of secondary degenerative disease, the potential advantages of a joint-preserving procedure must be weighed

against the high level of satisfaction associated with arthroplasty procedures.

## TREATMENT

### Conservative Management

Conservative management begins with an emphasis on early recognition of the underlying impingement disorder. The mainstay of treatment is identifying and modifying offending activities that precipitate symptoms. Some individuals can modify their lifestyles and stabilize the process for years. Efforts can be made to optimize mobility of the joint, but these are only modestly effective because motion is limited by the bony architecture, which cannot be corrected with manual techniques. Decompensatory disorders are those secondary problems that develop as individuals struggle to compensate for the chronic limitations imposed by the impingement. A conservative strategy must include assessment and treatment of the secondary problems, which can contribute substantially to the patient's symptoms.

For patients with degenerative disease, treatment may be lifestyle modifications to keep the symptoms manageable. For athletes pushing the joint beyond its diminished physiologic limitations, a specific program becomes more important. Optimizing core strength can aid in regaining the athlete's ability to compensate properly. Loading of a flexed hip can be particularly destructive in the presence of impingement; thus, repetitive training activities such as squats and lunges should be avoided or modified to limit hip flexion.

## Surgical Technique

The procedure begins with arthroscopy of the central compartment to assess for the pathology associated with cam impingement. This is carried out with the standard supine three-portal technique that has been well described in the literature (Fig. 4-8).[21-23] The characteristic feature of pathologic cam impingement is articular failure of the anterolateral acetabulum. The femoral head remains well preserved until late in the disease course. Early stages of the disease are characterized by closed grade I chondral blistering, which sometimes must be distinguished from normal articular softening. Our experience has been that most patients already have grade III or IV acetabular changes by the time of surgical intervention.[11] The articular surface is seen to separate or peel away from its attachment to the labrum (see

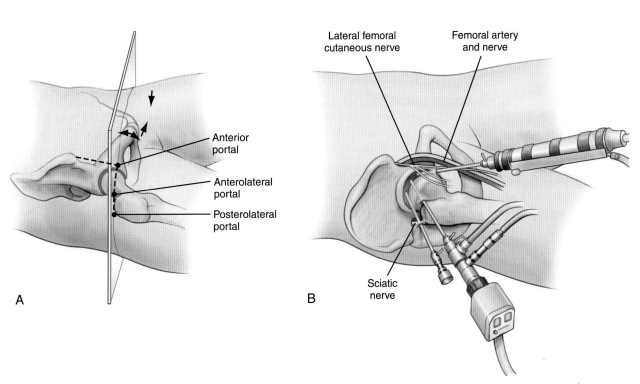

**FIGURE 4-8 A,** The site of the anterior portal coincides with the intersection of a sagittal line drawn distally from the anterior superior iliac spine and a transverse line across the superior margin of the greater trochanter. The direction of this portal courses approximately 45 degrees cephalad and 30 degrees toward the midline. The anterolateral and posterolateral portals are positioned directly over the superior aspect of the trochanter at its anterior and posterior borders. **B,** The relationship of the major neurovascular structures to the three standard portals is illustrated. The femoral artery and nerve lie well medial to the anterior portal. The sciatic nerve lies posterior to the posterolateral portal. The lateral femoral cutaneous nerve lies close to the anterior portal. Injury to this structure is avoided by using proper portal placement. The anterolateral portal is established first because it lies most centrally in the safe zone for arthroscopy. (**A** *courtesy of Smith & Nephew Endoscopy, Andover, Mass.*)

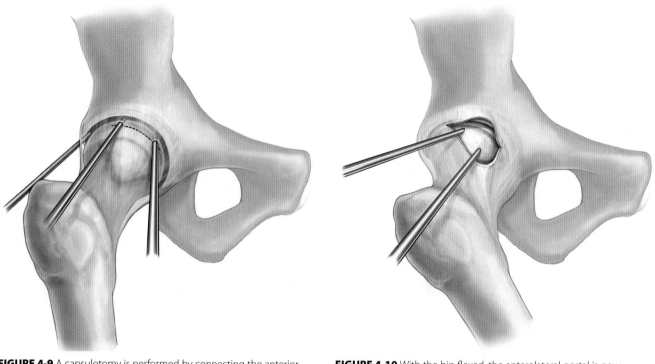

**FIGURE 4-9** A capsulotomy is performed by connecting the anterior and anterolateral portals (*dotted line*). This is geographically located adjacent to the area of the cam lesion. This capsulotomy is necessary so that the instruments can pass freely from the central to the peripheral compartment as traction is released and the hip is flexed.

**FIGURE 4-10** With the hip flexed, the anterolateral portal is now positioned along the neck of the femur. A cephalad (proximal) anterolateral portal has been placed. These two portals allow access to the entirety of the cam lesion in most cases. Their position also allows an unhindered view with the c-arm.

Fig. 4-16D); this is caused by the shear effect of the cam lesion. The labrum may be relatively well preserved but, with time, progressive fragmentation occurs. Often, the damaged articular surface of the labrum can be selectively débrided, preserving the capsular margin and potentially some of its labral seal function. If there is good-quality tissue that has been detached, repair can be performed with suture anchors. In cases of combined impingement with concomitant pincer lesions, the acetabulum is reshaped, either by takedown and subsequent refixation of the labrum or by débridement when the labral damage is advanced. The articular pathology is addressed with chondroplasty and microfracture as dictated by its severity.

After completing arthroscopy of the central compartment, the cam lesion is addressed from the peripheral compartment. A capsulotomy is created by connecting the anterior and anterolateral portals (Fig. 4-9). The posterolateral portal can be removed and the anterior and anterolateral cannulas are backed out of the central compartment. The traction is released and the hip is flexed approximately 35 degrees. As the hip is flexed under arthroscopic visualization, the line of demarcation between healthy femoral cartilage and abnormal fibrocartilage that covers the cam lesion can usually be identified.

A cephalad anterolateral portal is established approximately 5 cm above the anterolateral portal, entering through the capsulotomy that has already been established. These proximal and distal anterolateral portals work well for access-

ing and addressing the cam lesion (Fig. 4-10). The anterior portal can be removed or maintained if it is needed for better access to the medial side of the femoral neck.

Most of the work for performing the recontouring of the cam lesion (femoroplasty) lies in the soft tissue preparation. This includes capsular débridement, as necessary, to ensure complete visualization of the lesion and then removal of the fibrocartilage and scar that cover the abnormal bone (Fig. 4-11). With the hip flexed, the proximal portal provides better access for the lateral and posterior portion, whereas the distal portal is more anterior relative to the joint and provides the best access for the anterior part of the lesion. The lateral synovial fold is identified as the arthroscopic landmark for the retinacular vessels, and care is taken to preserve this structure during the recontouring (Fig. 4-12). Switching between the portals is important for full appreciation of the three-dimensional anatomy of the recontouring.

Once the bone has been fully exposed, recontouring is performed with a spherical burr. The goal is to remove the abnormal bone identified on the preoperative CT scan and re-create the normal concave relationship that should exist where the femoral neck meets the articular edge of the femoral head. It is best to begin by creating the line and depth of resection at the articular margin. The resection is then extended distally, tapering with the normal portion of the femoral head (Figs. 4-13 and 4-14). We recommend beginning the resection at the lateral posterior limit of the

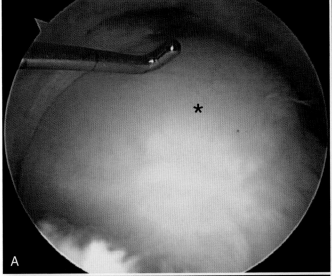

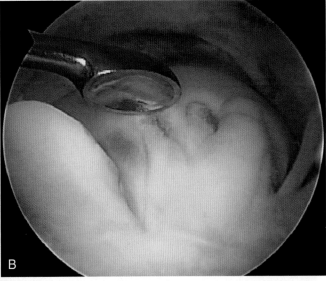

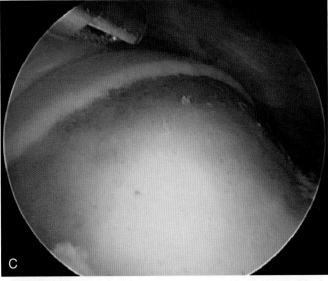

**FIGURE 4-11** The right hip is viewed from the anterolateral portal. **A,** The cam lesion is identified, covered in fibrocartilage (*asterisk*). **B,** An arthroscopic curette is used to denude the abnormal bone. **C,** The area to be excised has been fully exposed. The soft tissue preparation aids in precisely defining the margins to be excised.

**FIGURE 4-12** Viewed laterally, underneath the area of the lateral capsulotomy, the lateral synovial fold (*arrows*) is identified along the lateral base of the neck, representing the arthroscopic landmarks of the lateral retinacular vessels.

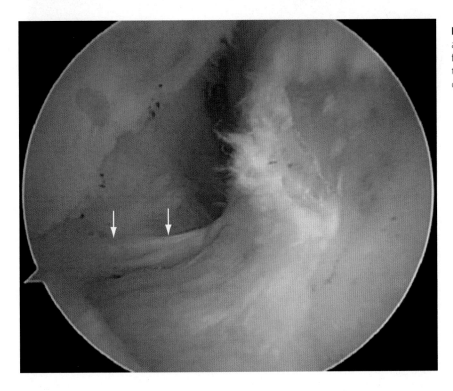

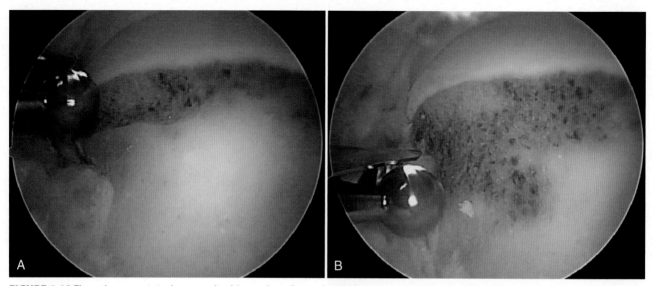

**FIGURE 4-13** The arthroscope is in the more distal (anterolateral) portal, with the instrumentation placed from the proximal portal. **A,** Bony resection is begun at the articular margin. **B,** The resection is then carried distally, re-creating the normal concave relationship.

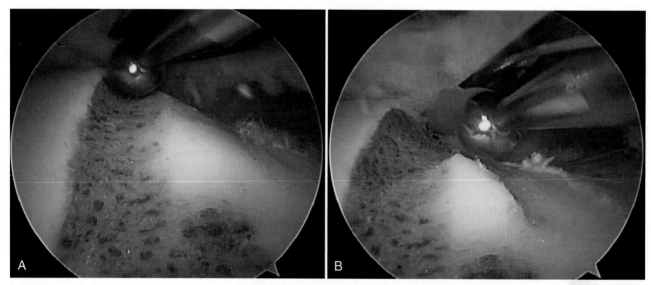

**FIGURE 4-14** The arthroscope is now in the proximal portal with the instrumentation introduced distally. **A,** The line of resection is continued along the anterior articular border of the bump. **B,** The recontouring is completed.

cam lesion, with the arthroscope in the more distal portal and instrumentation in the more proximal portal. The posterior extent of the resection is usually the most difficult; the resection is also the most critical to avoid notching the tensile surface of the femoral neck, and particular attention must be given to avoiding and preserving the lateral retinacular vessels. Then, switching the arthroscope to the proximal portal, the burr is introduced distally and the reshaping is completed along the anterior head and neck junc-

tion. Finally, attention is given to ensure that all bone debris is removed as thoroughly as possible to lessen the likelihood of developing heterotopic ossification. The quality of the recontouring is assessed and preservation of the lateral retinacular vessels is confirmed (Fig. 4-15).

Closure of the capsulotomy is not routinely performed. In cases in which instability might be a potential concern, such as dysplasia, the capsulotomy is limited and suture closure could be considered.

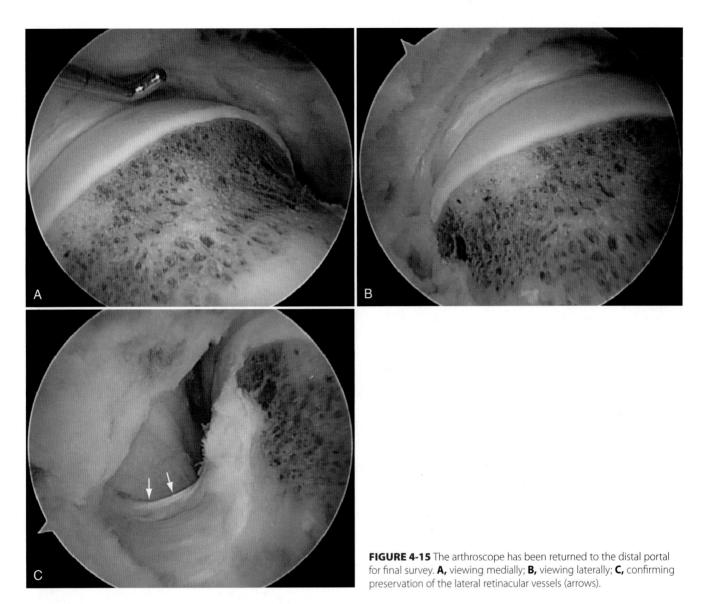

**FIGURE 4-15** The arthroscope has been returned to the distal portal for final survey. **A,** viewing medially; **B,** viewing laterally; **C,** confirming preservation of the lateral retinacular vessels (arrows).

## PEARLS & PITFALLS

- Be certain of the clinical relevance of the cam lesion. Radiographic evidence of cam morphology may often be encountered as an incidental finding. Make sure that the clinical findings indicate a hip problem and that the arthroscopic findings indicate pathology secondary to cam impingement.
- Make sure to complete the capsulotomy. A modest capsulotomy is necessary to mobilize the instruments adequately as they are moved from the central compartment with distraction to the peripheral compartment without distraction
- Fully expose the entirety of the cam lesion before beginning resection. Make sure to know the margins and amount of bone to be resected. This is important to avoid inadequate or excessive resection.
- Avoid reliance on fluoroscopic imaging in the absence of complete arthroscopic visualization during resection. This can result in erroneous bony resection.

- The first and most tedious step is the soft tissue preparation to expose the bone that needs to be resected. Bony resection should then proceed smoothly. Starting and stopping for added soft tissue exposure increases the risk of improper resection.
- Know the location of the lateral retinacular vessels. If in doubt, identify the vessels before beginning bony resection.
- Proper recontouring should entail a minimal risk for femoral neck fracture, but modest postoperative precautions are necessary. Weight bearing should be protected at least until good motor control of the hip musculature has been regained.
- Have a plan for assessing the amount of bone to remove whether this is based on visual templating of the abnormal bone from three-dimensional CT scans or on the intraoperative ROM to assess the adequacy of decompression. Note that the exact amount of bone to be removed, and the optimal method for assessing this, have not been defined. Inadequate or excessive resection are both problematic.

## Case Reports

### Case 1

A 20-year-old hockey player was evaluated, with a 4-year history of worsening right groin pain. Examination revealed diminished internal rotation of both hips (10 degrees). Forced flexion, adduction, and internal rotation of the right hip re-created the characteristic pain that he experienced with activities (Fig. 4-16).

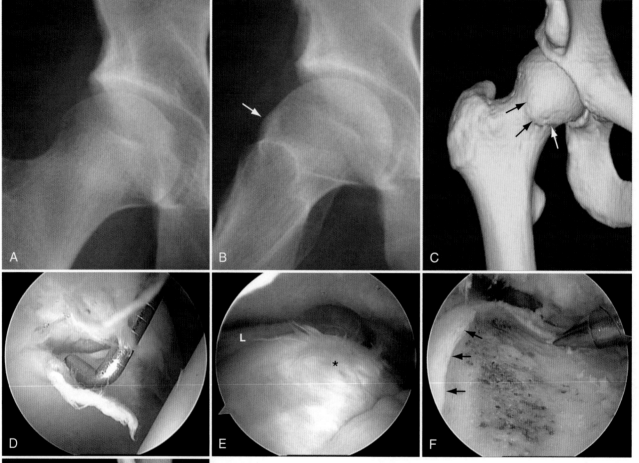

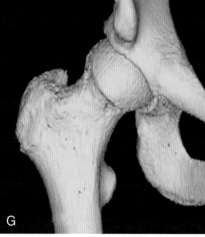

**FIGURE 4-16** Images of a 20-year-old hockey player with a 4-year history of right hip pain. **A,** AP radiograph is unremarkable. **B,** Frog-leg lateral radiograph demonstrates a morphologic variant with bony buildup at the anterior femoral head-neck junction (*arrow*) characteristic of cam impingement. **C,** Three-dimensional CT scan further defines the extent of the bony lesion (*arrows*). **D,** Viewing from the anterolateral portal, the probe introduced anteriorly displaces an area of articular delamination from the anterolateral acetabulum. This is characteristic of the peel-back mechanism created by the bony lesion shearing the articular surface during hip flexion. **E,** Viewed from the peripheral compartment, the bony lesion is identified (*asterisk*) immediately below the free edge of the acetabular labrum (L). **F,** The lesion has been excised, re-creating the normal concave relationship of the femoral head-neck junction immediately adjacent to the articular surface (*arrows*). Posteriorly, resection is limited to the midportion of the lateral neck to avoid compromising blood supply to the femoral head from the lateral retinacular vessels. **G,** A postoperative three-dimensional CT scan illustrates the extent of bony resection.

### Case 2

A 38-year-old woman presented with a 3-year history of progressively worsening pain and loss of motion of both hips, right worse than left. Symptoms were initially precipitated by horseback riding, but have now become troublesome with daily activities. Examination revealed an antalgic gait. Range of motion was restricted in both hips (35 degrees external rotation, 5 degrees internal rotation), with pain at all end ranges (Fig. 4-17).

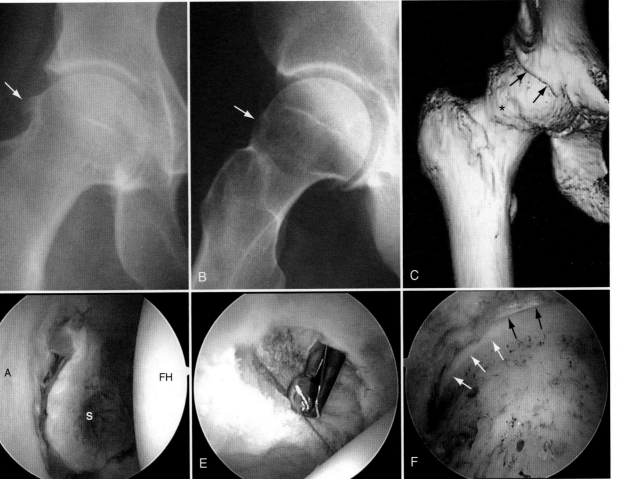

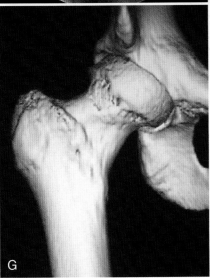

**FIGURE 4-17** Images of a 38-year-old woman with progressive pain and loss of motion of the right hip. **A,** AP radiograph demonstrates acquired bony buildup and osteophyte formation on the lateral femoral head (*arrow*). **B,** Frog-leg lateral radiograph further defines the bony buildup on the anterior femoral head (*arrow*). **C,** Three-dimensional CT scan further defines the femoral head osteophyte (*asterisk*) and anterior acetabular lesion (*arrows*). **D,** Arthroscopy of the central weight-bearing surface of the joint demonstrates good articular preservation of both the acetabulum (A) and femoral head (FH), with some reactive synovitis within the fossa (S). **E,** The anterior acetabular osteophyte is excised. **F,** Viewed peripherally, the femoral head has been recontoured showing the edge of the femoral articular surface (*white arrows*) and the labrum (*black arrows*). **G,** Postoperative three-dimensional CT scan demonstrates the extent of bony recontouring of both the acetabulum and femoral head.

## Case 3

A 15-year-old level 10 female gymnast presented with a 6-month history of left hip pain unresponsive to conservative treatment, including a protracted period of rest. Examination revealed a 20-degree loss of motion of the left hip compared with the right, with pain re-created on flexion, adduction, and internal rotation (Fig. 4-18).

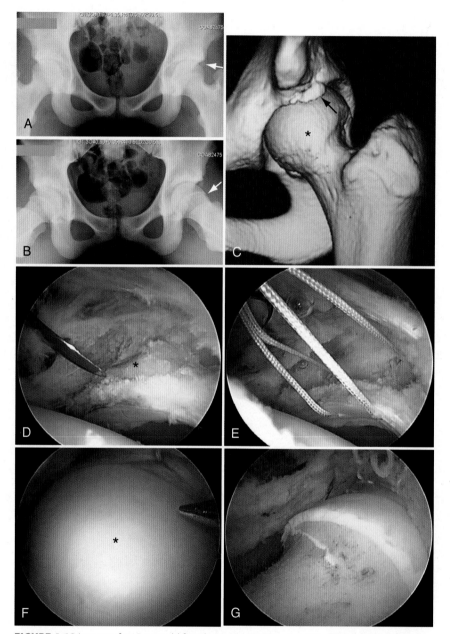

**FIGURE 4-18** Images of a 15-year-old female gymnast with pain and reduced internal rotation of the left hip. **A,** AP pelvic radiograph demonstrates a crossover sign of the left hip with an associated os acetabulum (*arrow*). **B,** Frog-leg lateral view illustrates asymmetrical cam lesion (*arrow*) present in the left hip and not the right. **C,** Three-dimensional CT scan further defines the pincer lesion with os acetabulum (*arrow*) and cam lesion (*asterisk*). **D,** Viewed from the anterolateral portal, the pincer lesion and os acetabulum (*asterisk*) are exposed, with the labrum being sharply released with an arthroscopic knife. **E,** The acetabular fragment has been removed and the rim trimmed with anchors placed for repair of the labrum. **F,** Viewed from the periphery, the cam lesion is identified (*asterisk*) covered in fibrocartilage. **G,** The cam lesion has been excised,  re-creating the normal concave contour of the head-neck junction adjacent to the site of labral refixation.

## POSTOPERATIVE PROTOCOL

### Rehabilitation

Formal supervised physical therapy begins within 1 or 2 days following surgery. An emphasis is on optimizing ROM, with early implementation of closed-chain joint stabilization and core strengthening exercises. The patient is allowed to bear weight as tolerated but crutches are used for 4 weeks as a precautionary measure to protect the femoroplasty site against any awkward twisting episodes. Once normal muscle tone and response patterns have been regained, these will adequately protect the joint from normal forces. Impact loading is avoided for 3 months while the bone fully remodels. The rehabilitation protocol is modified for microfracture by keeping the patient on strict, protected, weight-bearing status for 2 months. The patient is allowed to place the weight of the leg on the ground, which provides optimal neutralization of forces across the joint. Also, if a labral repair has been performed, excessive flexion and external rotation are avoided for the first 4 weeks.

A formal structured rehabilitation protocol is continued for 3 months. For athletes, functional progression is then advanced as tolerated. Although some athletes may resume unrestricted activities quickly, usually it is anticipated that another 1 to 3 months are necessary for full participation.

## OUTCOMES

We have reported on 200 patients (207 hips) with 100% follow-up at 1 to 2 years.[11] The average age was 33 years (range, 13 to 63 years). There were 138 males and 62 females, with 120 right and 87 left hips, and 163 patients underwent femoroplasty to correct cam impingement alone, whereas 44 patients underwent femoroplasty combined with correction of associated pincer impingement. Overall, the average improvement was 20 points (preoperative, 66; preoperative, 86). Using the Harris classification, 83% were improved, with 83% good and excellent results Viewing the results over time (see Fig. 4-8), continued improvement was noted throughout the first year, with results maintained in those with 2-year follow up. Most had Outerbridge grade IV (107) or grade III (83) articular damage on at least one side of the joint, and 58 underwent microfracture, with an average 20-point improvement (preoperative, 65; postoperative, 85). Comparing the results of cam and combined lesions, the results were comparable, with 20- versus 19-point improvement. The cam patients tended to be slightly younger, with an average age of 33 versus 35 years for combined lesions. A bimodal age distribution was identified, with a peak at age 20 and a second peak at age 43 years; 94 (45%) were sports-related. For those patients younger than 30 ($N = 88$), 62 (70%) were associated with athletic activities; after the third decade ($N = 119$), only 30 (25%) were associated with athletics. The under 30 group was also more male-dominated, with a male-to-female ratio of 3.1:1 compared with the over 30 group, with a male-to-female ratio of 1.9:1. One patient (0.5%) was converted to a total hip arthroplasty whereas 3 patients underwent a second arthroscopic procedure. There were three complications, but none were significant. There was one each of a transient neuro-praxia of the pudendal nerve and lateral femoral cutaneous nerve, which resolved uneventfully. One patient was incidentally noted to have developed heterotopic ossification within the capsule, which did not preclude a successful outcome.

In a more recent review, we identified a cohort of 163 athletes with cam-type FAI (141 isolated, 22 combined with pincer), in which there was a 100% minimum 1-year follow-up. The average age was 29 years, with 119 men and 44 women. There were 18 professional, 49 intercollegiate, and 96 high school or recreational athletes. The average improvement was 22 points (preoperative, 71; postoperative, 93), with 89% of professional and 90% of intercollegiate athletes returning to their previous level of athletic competition.

Other authors have reported outcomes of arthroscopic management of FAI specifically in regard to correction of the cam lesion. Ilizaliturri and colleagues have reported improvement in 16 of 19 patients (84%), with a minimum 2-year follow-up.[24] Bardakos and associates[25] have reported on femoral osteoplasty in 24 patients with 1-year follow-up compared with a control group in which arthroscopic débridement was performed without excising the impingement lesion. The modified Harris hip score was better in the study group (83) compared with the control group (77), and there was a significantly higher proportion of good to excellent results in the study group (83%) compared with the control group (60%). Brunner and coworkers[26] have reported on 45 athletically active individuals; 31 (69%) were able to resume their activities, with an average 2.4-year follow-up.

## SUMMARY

The arthroscope is instrumental in the treatment algorithm for cam impingement. Because cam morphology can exist in the absence of secondary associated joint pathology, the arthroscopic findings substantiate the need for correction of the underlying impingement. Most cases of cam impingement can be addressed arthroscopically. This is a technically demanding procedure that requires meticulous preparation for visualizing the cam lesion and careful orientation in recontouring of the bone to avoid inadequate or excessive resection. The results of the arthroscopic approach are at least comparable to those of the open method, with few complications. Successful results can be expected in most patients, including athletes and individuals seeking to return to an active lifestyle, with low morbidity.

## REFERENCES

1. Vulpius O, Stoffel A. *Orthopaadische Operationslehre*. Stuttgart, Germany: F. Enke; 1913.
2. Smith-petersen MN. Treatment of malum coxae senilis, old slipped upper femoral epiphysis, intrapelvic protrusion of the acetabulum, and coxa plana by means of acetabuloplasty. *J Bone Joint Surg Am*. 1936; 18:869-880.
3. Stulberg SD, Cordell LD, Harris WH, et al. Unrecognized childhood hip disease: a major cause of idiopathic osteoarthritis of the hip. In: Hip Society. *The Hip: Proceedings of the Third Open Scientific Meeting of the Hip Society*. St. Louis: Mosby; 1975.212-228.
4. Byrd JWT. Arthroscopy of select hip lesions. In: Byrd JWT, ed. *Operative Hip Arthroscopy*. New York: Thieme; 1998.153-170.

5. Byrd JWT. Hip arthroscopy: evolving frontiers. *Oper Tech Orthop.* 2004; 14:58-67 (Special Issue. Novel Techniques in Hip Surgery).

6. Myers SR, Eijer H, Ganz R. Anterior femoroacetabular impingement after periacetabular osteotomy. *Clin Orthop Relat Res.* 1999; (363):81-92.

7. Ganz R, Parvizi J, Beck M, et al. Femoroacetabular impingement. a cause for osteoarthritis in the hip. *Clin Orthop Relat Res.* 2003; (417):112-120.

8. Lavigne M, Parvizi J, Beck M, et al. Anterior femoroacetabular impingement. part I. Techniques of joint preserving surgery. *Clin Orthop Relat Res.* 2004;(418):61-66.

9. Byrd JWT. Hip morphology and related pathology. In: Johnson DH, Pedowitz RA, eds. *Practical Orthopaedic Sports Medicine and Arthroscopy.* Philadelphia: Lippincott, Williams & Wilkins; 2007.491-503.

10. Byrd JWT, Jones KS. Arthroscopic management of femoroacetabular impingement. *Instr Course Lect.* 2009; 58:231-239.

11. Byrd JWT, Jones KS. Arthroscopic "femoroplasty" in the management of cam-type femoroacetabular impingement. *Clin Orthop Relat Res.* 2009;(467):739-746.

12. Siebenrock KA, Wahab KHA, Werlen S, et al. Abnormal extension of the femoral head epiphysis as a cause of cam impingement. *Clin Orthop Relat Res.* 2004;(418):54-60.

13. Byrd JWT. Physical examination. In: Byrd JWT, ed. *Operative Hip Arthroscopy.* 2nd ed. New York: Springer; 2005.36-50.

14. Meyers WC, Foley DP, Garrett WE, et al. Management of severe lower abdominal or inguinal pain in high-performance athletes. PAIN (Performing Athletes with Abdominal or Inguinal Neuromuscular Pain Study Group). *Am J Sports Med.* 2000; 28:2-8.

15. Parvizi J, Leunig M, Ganz R. Femoroacetabular impingement. *J Am Acad Orthop Surg.* 2007; 15:561-570.

16. Meyer DC, Beck M, Ellis T, et al. Comparison of six radiographic projections to assess femoral head/neck asphericity. *Clin Orthop Relat Res.* 2006;(445):181-185.

17. Notzli H, Wyss TF, Stoecklin CH, et al. The contour of the femoral head/neck junction as a predictor for the risk of anterior impingement. *J Bone Joint Surg Br.* 2002; 84:556-560.

18. Byrd JWT, Jones KS. Diagnostic accuracy of clinical assessment, MRI, gadolinium MRI, and intra-articular injection in hip arthroscopy patients. *Am J Sports Med.* 2004; 32:1668-1674.

19. Philippon MJ. Schenker ML. Arthroscopy for the treatment of femoroacetabular impingement in the athlete. *Clin Sports Med.* 2006; 25:299-308.

20. Tonnis D, Heinecke A. Acetabular and femoral anteversion. relationship with osteoarthritis of the hip. *J Bone Joint Surg Am.* 1999; 81:1747-1770.

21. Byrd JWT. Hip arthroscopy utilizing the supine position. *Arthroscopy.* 1994; 10(3).275-280.

22. Byrd JWT. The supine approach. In: Byrd JWT, ed. *Operative Hip Arthroscopy.* 2nd ed. New York: Springer; 2005.145-169.

23. Byrd JWT. Hip arthroscopy by the supine approach. *Instr Course Lect.* 2006; 55:325-336.

24. Ilizaliturri VM, Orozco-Rodriguez L, Acosta-Rodriguez E, Camacho-Galindo J. Arthroscopic treatment of cam-type femoroacetabular impingement. *J Arthroplasty.* 2008;23:226-234.

25. Bardakos NV, Vasconcelos JC, Villar RN. Early outcome of hip arthroscopy for femoroacetabular impingement. the role of femoral osteoplasty in symptomatic improvement. *J Bone Joint Surg Br.* 2008; 90:1570-1575.

26. Brunner A, Horisberger M, Herzog RF. Sports and recreation activity of patients with femoroacetabular impingement before and after arthroscopic osteoplasty. *Am J Sports Med.* 2009; 37:917-922.

# Femoroacetabular Impingement: Pincer

Marc J. Philippon ● Bruno G. Schroder e Souza

Femoroacetabular impingement (FAI) was first reported over 70 years ago.[1] However, it was not until recently was it described as a cause of hip osteoarthritis.[2-4] Multiple forms of proximal femur and acetabular dysplasias have been described,[5-7] but two specific mechanisms of lesion are acknowledged as being responsible for FAI, cam and pincer. Cam impingement occurs when an abnormally shaped femoral head contacts a normal acetabulum, particularly during flexion and internal rotation. Pincer impingement involves a normal femoral head contacting an abnormally shaped, deep, or retroverted acetabulum. The patterns of intra-articular soft-tissue injury resulting from the impingement appear to be unique to the distinct type of deformity.[8]

In cam impingement, the "bump" at the femoral head-neck junction produces a shearing force, displacing the labrum toward the capsule and the adjacent articular cartilage into the joint.[2,8] Softening of the articular cartilage can be observed as a wave sign when arthroscopically probed before frank chondral delamination.[9] With repeated insults, the labrum may completely detach from the acetabular rim, and the cartilage may fully delaminate (Fig. 5-1).

In pincer impingement, the labrum is essentially trapped between the bony structures; thus, it often bruises and flattens.[2,8] With persistent pincer impingement, the labrum may degenerate, with cyst formation or ossification of the fibrocartilage. Persistent pincer impingement may lead to a chondral defect (a contrecoup lesion) at the posteroinferior acetabulum or posteromedial femoral head. The chondral injuries resulting from a pincer impingement are typically less severe than those resulting from a cam impingement (Fig. 5-2).

Demographically, cam impingement seems to be more common in young male athletes and pincer impingement in female athletes.[2,10,11] Cam and pincer impingement rarely occur in isolation, and the combination has been termed *mixed cam-pincer impingement*. With this disorder, an abnormal femoral head or head-neck junction articulates with an abnormal acetabulum. In one epidemiologic study of 149 hips with impingement, 26 (17.4%) had isolated cam impingement, 16 (10.7%) had isolated pincer impingement, and 107 (71.8%) had combined cam-pincer impingement.[8]

In this chapter, we are going to describe the clinical and radiologic presentation of pincer deformity and our current surgical approach to that condition.

## CLINICAL PRESENTATION

Pincer impingement may be caused by general acetabular overcoverage (coxa profunda) or acetabular retroversion and has been shown to be associated with osteoarthritis of the hip.[2-4,7] During flexion of the hip, the edge of the anterior wall and the anterosuperior roof of a retroverted acetabulum are vulnerable to impingement because they tend to lie directly in the path of the femoral neck.

Reynolds and colleagues[7] have described the clinical presentation of acetabular retroversion. In this condition, there is not necessarily any change in the range of movement of the hip. When the retroversion is marked, however, there is a demonstrable alteration in the pattern of hip flexion in the neutral line. This may be limited to as little as 90 degrees, progressing to a full range only when allowed to move simultaneously into external rotation and abduction in a Drehman sign–like pattern.[12,13] The contact of the femoral neck to the edge of the acetabulum on

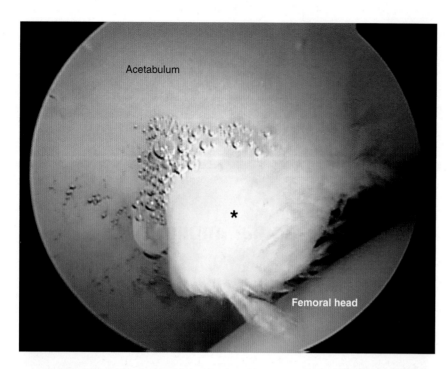

**FIGURE 5-1** Chondral delamination in the anterior-superior aspect of the acetabulum is common in cam impingement. *, chondral flap.

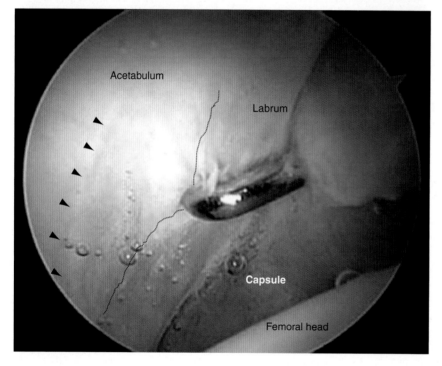

**FIGURE 5-2** Partial labral tear in the anterior aspect of the right acetabulum (*line*) being probed. A flattened and yellowish labrum is usually seen in isolated pincer deformity. Chondral lesions (*arrowheads*) are often observed in the periphery of the acetabulum and are less severe than those observed in cam deformities.

maximum flexion and the need to contour its retroverted mouth to continue the full range of motion explains that phenomenon.[7] In these individuals, the limb tends to lie at rest in a position externally rotated at the hip. The range of external rotation, especially in the flexed position, is more generous than usual, often exceeding 60 degrees. The range of internal rotation may be limited proportionally. Asked to sit on the floor, such patients are comfortable only with their hips flexed, abducted, and externally rotated. Some describe a dislike of sitting in a chair with legs crossed, especially with the symptomatic leg crossed over the other. In some cases of coxa profunda, abduction may be limited by the lateral impingement of the femoral neck to the acetabulum.[14]

In the early presentation, the impingement test usually will elicit discomfort felt in the groin.[7,15-17] The onset of the symptoms may be related to a new athletic activity, and females seem to be particularly susceptible. The pain is often intermittent and exacerbated by an excessive demand on hip flexion, such as occurs with athletic activities and in very flexible hips. In many cases, individuals take part in athletic activities or have occupations in which some discomfort is accepted as part of the activity. For that reason, a delayed diagnosis is not uncommon.[7] Despite the recent attention directed to this condition, some patients have even had surgery in other sites because of a missed diagnosis.

The late presentation will be found in the age range of 30 to 50 years.[7] Usually, the patient will remember few or no troublesome symptoms from their younger years, but direct questioning may reveal otherwise. In the impingement test, passive internal rotation induces shear forces at the labrum and will create a sharp pain when there is a labral and/or chondral lesion.[2,15-18] Patients with impingement can have pain with athletic activities and even while sitting with the hip extremely flexed. Mechanical symptoms and limitations to athletic and daily activities may be present; these usually indicate intra-articular soft-tissue damage related to the impingement.[11] Degenerative signs may predominate after a prolonged time without treatment.[19,20]

## IMAGING

Pincer impingement is the result of overcoverage of the hip. It is commonly associated with acetabular protrusion, coxa profunda, or a retroverted acetabulum.[7] Pincer impingement is also the result of a linear contact between the acetabular rim and femoral head-neck junction because of general or focal acetabular overcoverage (Fig. 5-3).[7,13]

Normally, general acetabular overcoverage is correlated with the radiologic depth of the acetabular fossa. A normal hip appears on an anteroposterior pelvic radiograph with the acetabular fossa line lying laterally to the ilioischial line. A coxa profunda is defined with the floor of the acetabular fossa touching or overlapping the ilioischial line medially. Protrusio acetabuli occurs when the femoral head is overlapping the ilioischial line medially. Both forms relate to an increased depth of the acetabulum; however, at this stage, no clear information exists that the two entities are a continuation of each other.[13] Generally, a deep acetabulum is associated with excessive acetabular coverage that can be quantified with the lateral center edge angle or the acetabular index.[20] Another parameter for quantification of femoral coverage is the femoral head extrusion index.[21]

An additional observation on plain radiographs may be juxta-articular fibrocystic changes (herniation pits) at the anterosuperior aspect of the femoral neck.[22]

The lateral center edge angle is the angle formed by a vertical line and a line connecting the femoral head center with the lateral edge of the acetabulum. A normal lateral center edge angle varies between 25 (which defines a dysplasia)[20] and 39 degrees (which is an indicator for acetabular overcoverage).[6]

The acetabular index is the angle formed by a horizontal line and a line connecting the medial point of the sclerotic zone with the lateral center of the acetabulum. In hips with coxa profunda or protrusio acetabuli, the acetabular index (also called the acetabular roof angle) is typically 0 degree or even negative.[13]

The femoral head extrusion index defines the percentage of femoral head that is uncovered when a horizontal line is drawn parallel to the interteardrop line.[21] A normal extrusion index is less than 25%[23]; however, to our knowledge, no study has defined a minimum extrusion.[13]

Focal acetabular overcoverage can occur in the anterior or the posterior part of the acetabulum. Anterior overcoverage is called cranial acetabular retroversion or anterior focal acetabular retroversion; it causes anterior femoroacetabular impingement that can be reproduced clinically with painful flexion and internal rotation.[7] By careful tracing on an anteroposterior (AP) pelvis radiograph, the anterior and posterior acetabular rims can be identified. A normal acetabulum is anteverted and has the anterior rim line projected medially to the posterior wall line. To distinguish between a too prominent anterior wall and a deficient posterior wall, the posterior wall must be depicted in more detail. These situations can be distinguished by the crossover sign, the ischial spine sign and the posterior wall sign.[13,24]

A focal overcoverage of the anterosuperior acetabulum causes a cranially retroverted acetabulum. This is defined with the anterior rim line being lateral to the posterior rim in the cranial part of the acetabulum and crossing the latter in the distal part of the acetabulum. This figure-of-eight configuration is called the crossover sign.[7]

The posterior wall sign was introduced as an indicator for a prominent posterior wall. This can cause posterior impinge-

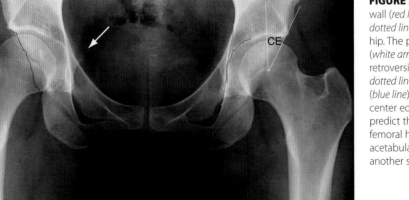

**FIGURE 5-3** In this image, the posterior acetabular wall (*red line*) intersects the anterior wall (*blue dotted line*), forming the crossover sign on the right hip. The prominent ischial spine into the pelvis (*white arrow*) is another sign of acetabular retroversion. On the left hip, the acetabulum (*red dotted line*) projects medially to the ilioischial line (*blue line*), which is defined as coxa profunda. The center edge (CE) angle is another parameter to predict the depth of the socket. The center of the femoral head is located laterally to the posterior acetabular wall, as illustrated on the left hip, is another sign of acetabular retroversion.

ment with reproducible pain in hip extension and external rotation. In a normal hip, the visible outline of the posterior rim descends approximately through the center point of the femoral head. If the posterior line lies laterally to the femoral center, a more prominent posterior wall is present. In contrast, a deficient posterior wall has the posterior rim medial to the femoral head center.[7] A deficient posterior wall is often correlated with acetabular retroversion or dysplasia,[23] and an excessive posterior wall can often be seen in hips with coxa profunda or protrusio acetabuli but can also occur as an isolated entity.

The ischial spine sign consists of a pre-eminent projection of that structure to the pelvis on an AP radiograph. It denotes not only global acetabular retroversion, but also the involvement of the whole hemipelvis in the deformity.[24]

The common use for computed tomography (CT) scans in the evaluation of impingement is to allow three-dimensional reconstruction of the hip joint for detailed definition of femoral head-neck asphericities and reduced offset, which cause osseous impingement, as well as determination of the version of the femoral neck and acetabulum.[25,26] Magnetic resonance imaging (MRI) is useful to assess labral injury and the articular cartilage and to evaluate concomitant conditions.[26]

## TECHNIQUE

### Surgical Setup

Arthroscopy of the hip can be performed with the patient in a lateral or supine position.[27,28] Our preference is the modified supine approach.[29] We recommend a combination of general anesthesia with a lumbar plexus sciatic regional block for complete muscular paralysis.[30] After the induction of anesthesia, the patient is positioned on a standard fracture table that allows independent lower extremity traction.

### Portal Placement

Accurate portal placement is essential for optimal visualization of all intra-articular structures and safe access to the hip joint. We used to do three portals to perform FAI surgeries—the anterolateral, anterior, and distal lateral accessory portals.[31] Currently, we think that for most cases, only the anterolateral (lateral paratrochanteric) and midanterior portals are required.[10]

The anterolateral portal is referenced off the greater trochanter. This portal is placed approximately 1 to 2 cm superior to the tip of the greater trochanter and 1 to 2 cm anterior from this proximal point. The needle is guided slightly cephalic and posterior to converge along the direction of the femoral neck, at an angle of approximately 15 to 20 degrees in relation to the floor.

The midanterior portal is placed approximately 7 cm distal and medial to the anterolateral portal, in a line subtending about 45 degrees with the longitudinal axis of the leg. This entry point is less likely to cause injury to the lateral cutaneous femoral nerve and provides a good angle for anchor insertion in the acetabulum and to approach the peripheral compartment. The needle is inserted aiming proximally and medially, so that it penetrates the capsule under direct visualization of the arthroscope in the center of the anterior triangle formed by the labrum, femoral head, and capsule (Fig. 5-4).[10,29,30]

**FIGURE 5-4** The midanterior portal (right hip) is established under direct visualization of the triangle formed by the femoral head, labrum, and capsule.

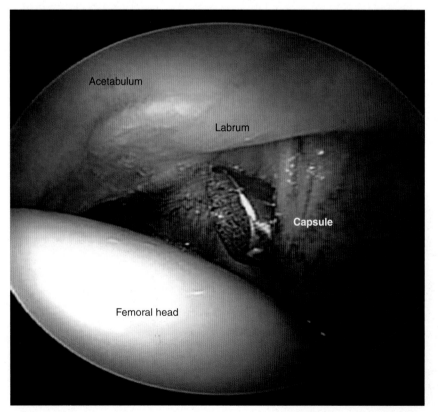

## Joint Inspection

At this point, a complete inspection of the central compartment must be performed. A group of specialists recently developed a geographic zone system to describe and record the surgical findings,[32] although the clock system has been used in many studies.[10,11,27,29,31,33-35] The identification of anatomic landmarks (e.g., stellate crease, transverse ligament, synovial folds) help guide the location and amount of bone resection that will be later performed.

On joint entry, a systematic examination should be performed of the entire acetabular labrum. The fibrocartilaginous labrum is normally adhered to the acetabular rim and transitions to the hyaline articular cartilage in a zone of approximately 1 to 2 mm.[36] The labrum is widest anteriorly and thickest superiorly, corresponding to the weight-bearing region of the acetabulum.[37] The labrum has been shown to provide approximately 5 mm of additional femoral head coverage and primarily functions as a physiologic joint seal.[38] A torn labrum is thought to alter load transmission in the joint and increase articular cartilage consolidation.[38] In our practice, we have observed five types of labral tears—detached, midsubstance longitudinal, flap, frayed, and degenerative. Chondral lesions may be cartilage softening, fraying, or fissuring, subchondral cysts, chondral flaps, or full-thickness abrasion with subchondral bone exposure.[16]

In patients with pincer lesions, the most common finding is a bruised, flattened, and degenerative labrum caused by abutment against the femoral neck.[8,39] Intrasubstance labral cysts and labral ossification may occur.[2] Labral ossification accounts for additional acetabular overhanging and may contribute to the impingement. In pincer lesions, a more circumferential pattern of labral and chondral damages was found compared with cam lesions. It has been reported that chondral lesions may occur from 7 to 5 o'clock in the right hip (zones 1 to 5), but most of the lesions are encountered from 12 to 2 o'clock in the right hip (zones 2 and 3).[40] Nevertheless, those lesions tend to be less severe and are concentrated on the periphery of the joint (watershed zone). The area of chondral lesion often delineates the area with excessive bone overhang. Experimental studies in cadavers predicted a lack of accuracy in resection of acetabular bone by arthroscopic rim-trimming procedure of about 19 degrees,[35] but those studies were performed in specimens without pincer deformity and therefore lacked this important intraoperative sign to help in the arthroscopic orientation of the bone resection.

Another typical intra-articular finding in pincer deformities is the posterior-inferior chondral lesion in the acetabulum, sometimes accompanied by a kissing lesion on the femoral head, known as a contrecoup lesion.[2] The attributed cause for these injuries is a leverage of the femoral neck against the anterior margin of the acetabulum, leading to posterior dislocation of the hip mechanism, with a chondral lesion in the area under shear stress.

## Capsulotomy

After thorough inspection, capsulotomy is performed about 1 cm distal to the labral margin. The extension of the capsulotomy will depend on the ability to maneuver the instruments to perform all the necessary procedures.[30] The procedure usually consists of performing the capsulotomy from the correspondent area of the anterolateral portal in the capsule to the midanterior portal. Although preserving the iliofemoral ligament by avoiding excessive anterior extension of the capsulotomy anteriorly is desired, this should not impede adequate exposure and instrumentation. Therefore, further extension of the capsulotomy anteriorly and posteriorly is allowed as long as the ligament is repaired afterward.[10] At all stages, the capsulotomy should be performed under direct visualization. It should be noted that the lateral retinacular vessels that provide an important source of blood supply to the femoral head lie under the lateral synovial fold, and would be at risk if blind transection were performed too laterally.[33,41]

After capsulotomy, two strategies are possible, depending on the labral condition and amount of acetabular bone resection required. Both rim trimming with and without labral takedown can be performed and will be described separately.

## Rim Trimming with Labral Takedown

In there is labral detachment at its base, which is particularly common in cases with associated cam impingement, the labrum should be separated in the watershed zone so that the underlying bone deformity can be corrected and the labrum reattached with suture anchors.[30] First, we delineate the chondrolabral junction by controlled application of a monopolar radiofrequency (RF) chisel. This will contract the fibrocartilage and better define the tear, preventing sacrifice of healthy labral tissue and stabilizing the adjacent acetabular cartilage. Any chondral flaps are removed after demarcation with the aid of the same RF device. The area between the labrum and capsule is dissected with a shaver and the labrum is completely detached from the acetabular rim as much as is needed. The acetabular bony overhang responsible for the pincer deformity can be removed with a motorized burr before or after complete labral detachment, depending on the amount of resection required (Figs. 5-5 and 5-6). The amount should be determined preoperatively by analysis of the imaging studies. There is a correlation between the center edge (CE) angle and the amount of lateral resection in millimeters. The resection should allow a postoperative CE angle of at least 25 degrees.[42] The working portal to perform most of the resection is the lateral portal, although switching portals is essential for complete assessment of the resection.

### Labral Reattachment

The acetabular rim, now reshaped, is the ideal site at which to reattach the labrum. A bleeding cancellous bed has been

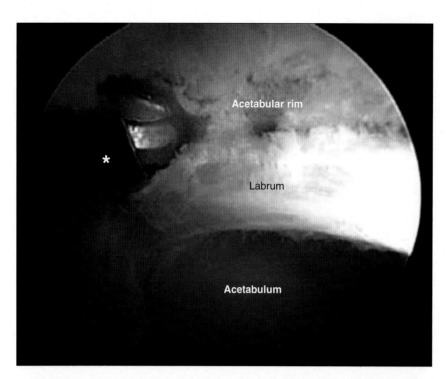

**FIGURE 5-5** Acetabular rim trimming with an arthroscopic burr (*) can be performed before labral takedown.

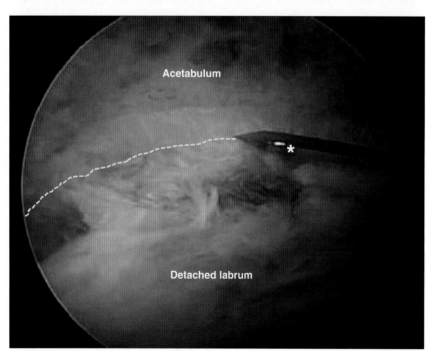

**FIGURE 5-6** Labral detachment with an arthroscopic blade (*) viewed from the peripheral compartment, after acetabular rim trimming. The limit between the articular cartilage and acetabular labrum is observed (*yellow dashed line*).

reported as necessary for labral refixation because of the relatively avascular nature of the labrum.[43] Experimental studies have demonstrated that it can heal directly to the bone, as well as to the surrounding capsule.[44] The acetabular rim provides solid fixation for the anchors and a stable base to allow for labral repair. We use one bioabsorbable 2.9-mm anchor for every 1 cm of labral detachment. Smaller patients might require 2.3-mm anchors. More anchors should be placed, as needed, to provide good stability and shape to the labrum so that it can exert its physiologic functions.[10,11]

The anchors are placed about 2 mm off the acetabular rim in the area of the rim trimming under direct visualization of the entry point and adjacent articular surface (Fig. 5-7).[30] In general, the anterolateral portal allows the insertion of anchors in the superolateral aspect of the acetabulum, where most of the lesions are found. Because the guide sleeve is directed to the trimmed acetabular margin in a divergent direction to avoid intra-articular penetration, a cranial angle of about 45 degrees is often observed in the coronal plane. The direction in the transverse plane for placement of anchors at

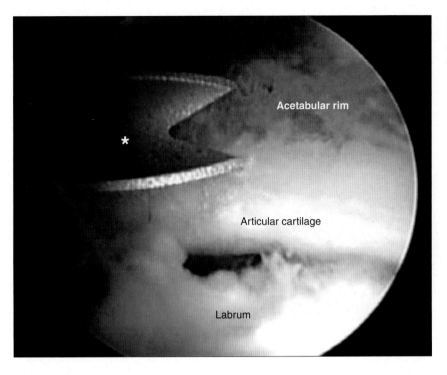

**FIGURE 5-7** The guide for the anchor drill (*) must be placed about 1 to 2 mm from the articular surface and be directed divergent to the joint to avoid articular penetration.

the 12 o'clock position (zone 3) in the acetabulum is parallel to the ground. As more anterior placements are necessary, a forward inclination of the guide is performed. The limit for that is usually the position corresponding to 2 o'clock (considering the right acetabulum), where the insertion angle may be too acute. For the insertion of anterior-most anchors (beyond the 2 o'clock position, or zone 1), the midanterior portal should be used. Fluoroscopy may be used during the procedure to ensure optimal placement.

We recommend tapping the sleeve slightly into the acetabular rim and after drilling the anchor path, manually driving anchor into place using tactile sensation as a guide.[30] While drilling, it is critical to visualize the articular surface of the acetabulum to ensure that it is not being compromised. If bulging of the articular surface is noted, the angle of the anchor must be redirected. Once the anchor it is in place, the articular surface should again be visualized to verify that it has not been penetrated (Fig. 5-8).

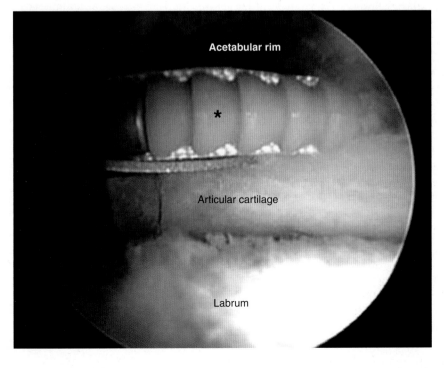

**FIGURE 5-8** A bioabsorbable anchor is placed (*) and the articular surface is checked to ensure that no bulging has occurred.

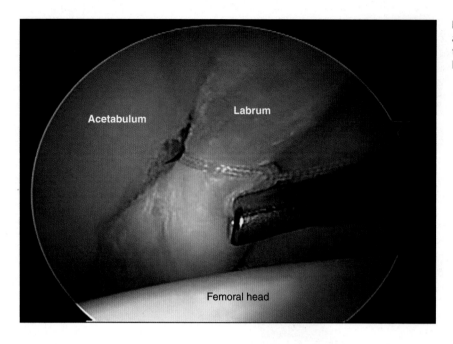

**FIGURE 5-9** The labrum is reattached with arthroscopic sliding knots. For better tensioning, the traction may be released while the knot is being tied.

A clear 8.25-mm cannula is then introduced through the working portal and the sutures are drawn back through it. It can be also inserted before the anchor delivery device. However, in more extreme positions, it may hinder the mobility of the guide. The next step is to deliver a limb of suture between the labrum and acetabular rim with a suture passer. As the suture is pulled out through the clear cannula, it is important to visualize the anchor to ensure that the correct suture limb is being retrieved. The cannula must then be pulled back slightly for improved visualization, and the suture is tied down using standard arthroscopic knot-tying technique. In some cases, traction may be released while it is being tied to get better knot fixation (Figs. 5-8 and 5-9).

A translabral suture stitch may be done in a thick labrum (on the weight-bearing zone) to provide better apposition. In that case, one limb of the suture is delivered intra-articularly between the labrum and acetabular rim. The labrum is pierced with the suture passer in its midsubstance in an outside-in direction and a loop of the intra-articular limb of the suture is pulled through it. The suture passer is removed from the labrum and is used to pull the free end of the same suture limb completely through the loop, retrieving it through the cannula. At this point, as both limbs of the suture are tensioned simultaneously, the labrum gets closer to the acetabular rim, allowing a suture-free margin of it to be in contact with the femoral head. The suture is then tied using standard arthroscopic knot-tying technique (Fig. 5-10).

## Rim Trimming Without Labral Takedown

In rare cases without labral tear and in which a minimum amount of acetabular bone resection is required, the rim trimming can be performed without labral takedown.[10,45] Most of those cases are accompanied by cam deformities and we use the following surgical strategy.

To obtain adequate space to work between the capsule and labrum, we release traction, extend the capsulotomy, and treat the peripheral compartment first. We use a shaver to dissect the space between the capsule and labrum, exposing the underlying bone. The resection is then performed as planned. Traction is introduced again and the labrum is inspected. Unless a very modest resection was performed (1 mm), the chondrolabral junction usually is torn or so thin that an additional attachment to the acetabular rim is necessary. It is our impression that the junction is not able to handle the physiologic stresses when the supportive bone to the labrum has been removed. Failure in the watershed zone is to be expected when it is the only attachment of the labrum. In fact, the senior author (MJP) has revised one case in which that procedure was performed without additional fixation of the labrum to the bone; the intraoperative findings were labral tear at the transition (watershed) zone and adherence of the labrum to the adjacent capsule, despite no history of new trauma. Therefore, we currently perform and recommend anchor placement and suture fixation of the labrum to the acetabulum in those situations, despite not taking down the labrum. Additional studies are required to establish whether this precaution should be taken. However, we think that this practice at least allows a more active rehabilitation process, which we believe is very important to prevent adherences and allow early return to most activities.[46]

The technique for anchor placement without labral detachment does not differ much from that described for the other. It may be slightly more difficult to inspect the entry point and articular surface constantly during anchor insertion. The suture fixation follows the same technique, except that the chondrolabral junction must be pierced to pass one of the suture limbs between the labrum and acetabulum.

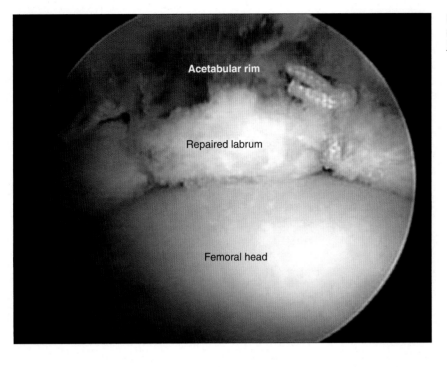

**FIGURE 5-10** The repaired labrum must be stable and provide an adequate sealing effect to the joint.

## Other Lesions and Completing the Procedure

Peripheral chondral lesions, usually related to pincer lesion, often disappear after the resection of the underlying pathologic bone. The remaining chondral edge then needs to be stabilized; a flexible RF probe may be used for that purpose and to contour the edges of the labrum. However, more extensive chondral damage may be present, mainly when other conditions are associated or the treatment was performed long after the onset of symptoms. In those cases, local débridement, thermal chondroplasty, or microfractures may be performed, depending on the lesion type.[10,47]

It is important to note that isolated pincer lesions occur in only 10.7% of the cases.[8] Femoral deformities usually coexist and should be addressed to prevent failure of the treatment.[48] After all lesions are treated, dynamic inspection of the joint, without traction must be done arthroscopically to disclose any possible conflict between the labrum and femoral neck. Any signs of impingement should elicit further bone reshaping or labral contouring. The need for more anchors is commonly noted at this time.[10] We always test all the possible movements related to patient activities to obtain maximum range of motion without impingement (Fig. 5-11). Dynamic

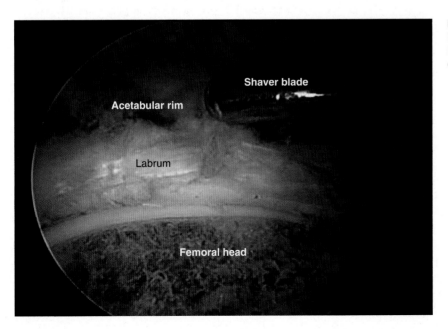

**FIGURE 5-11** Final appearance of a repaired labrum after femoral osteoplasty and rim trimming. In the dynamic examination, there should be no conflict between the femoral neck and labrum.

fluoroscopy may aid in determining the adequacy of bone resection, but is not a substitute for direct arthroscopic inspection. Following dynamic visualization, we close the capsule, which we believe to be important to resume rehabilitation and prevent instability.[49]

---

### PEARLS & PITFALLS

**SURGICAL SETUP**

**Pearls**

Complete patient relaxation, use of a well-padded perineal post, and control of traction time are paramount to prevent complications related to traction.

Alternating work between the peripheral and central compartments helps decrease the amount of continuous traction time.

**RIM TRIMMING WITH LABRAL TAKEDOWN**

**Pearl**

The use of an RF device to delineate the limit of the chondrolabral junction helps prevent the sacrifice of healthy labral tissue and helps stabilize adjacent acetabular cartilage

**LABRAL REATTACHMENT**

**Pearls**

Although 2.9-mm anchors usually provide the best purchase, smaller anchors may be necessary, especially at the thinner portions of the acetabular wall (3 and 9 o'clock).

Translabral sutures may be used in thicker portions of the labrum when the objective is to minimize labral eversion.

**Pitfalls**

In patients with coxa vara, the anterolateral portal usually remains relatively more proximal to the acetabular rim. Failure to incline the guide proximally will lead to intra-articular penetration of the anchor.

Inappropriate entry point and guide angulation may lead to intra-articular penetration of the anchor, chondral damage, and/or inadequate fixation

**RIM TRIMMING WITHOUT LABRAL TAKEDOWN**

**Pitfall**

After rim trimming without labral takedown, repair with anchors is often necessary to prevent abnormal labral mobility and consequent failure at the watershed zone.

**OTHER LESIONS AND COMPLETING THE PROCEDURE**

**Pearl**

Dynamic examination under arthroscopic visualization is the best way to obtain full decompression of the impingement.

---

## REHABILITATION

Rehabilitation following arthroscopic femoroacetabular impingement treatment includes restrictions of weight bearing, rotation, and movement. Patients are kept at 20 lb of weight bearing with 8 to 12 hours daily of continuous passive movement (CPM) for 4 weeks. An antirotation bolster to prevent external hip rotation of the hip is used for 10 days after surgery.[10,30,46,49] Microfracture treatment of chondral lesions involves 6 to 8 weeks of partial weight bearing and continued CPM.[47] Physiotherapy is used first to restore passive motion, followed by active motion and then strengthening exercises. Internal rotation is gained first, and then external rotation. We also recommend passive hip pendulums or circumduction movements to prevent adhesion formation.

## SUMMARY

In conclusion, this approach to treat pincer lesions resembles those previously described to trim the acetabular rim and repair the labrum, with some modifications.[31] Our current approach has resulted from experience treating over 2000 patients with FAI arthroscopically, and it has shown to be efficient and reproducible.[10]

## REFERENCES

1. Smith-Petersen MN. Treatment of malum coxae senilis, old slipped upper femoral epiphysis, intrapelvic protrusion of the acetabulum, and coxa plana by means of acetabuloplasty. *J Bone Joint Surg.* 1936;18:869-880.
2. Ganz R, Parvizi J, Beck M, et al. Femoroacetabular impingement: a cause for osteoarthritis of the hip. *Clin Orthop Relat Res.* 2003; (417):112-120.
3. Ganz R, Leunig M, Leunig-Ganz K, Harris WH. The etiology of osteoarthritis of the hip: an integrated mechanical concept. *Clin Orthop Relat Res.* 2008;466:264-272.
4. Giori NJ, Trousdale RT. Acetabular retroversion is associated with osteoarthritis of the hip. *Clin Orthop Relat Res.* 2003;(417): 263-269.
5. Tönnis D. *Congenital Dysplasia and Dislocation of the Hip in Children and Adults.* Berlin: Springer; 1987.
6. Tönnis D, Heinecke A. Acetabular and femoral anteversion: relationship with osteoarthritis of the hip. *J Bone Joint Surg Am.* 1999;81:1747-1770.
7. Reynolds D, Lucas J, Klaue K. Retroversion of the acetabulum. A cause of hip pain. *J Bone Joint Surg Br.* 1999;81:281-288.
8. Beck M, Kalhor M, Leunig M, Ganz R. Hip morphology influences the pattern of damage to the acetabular cartilage: femoroacetabular impingement as a cause of early osteoarthritis of the hip. *J Bone Joint Surg Br.* 2005;87:1012-1018.
9. Johnston TL, Schenker ML, Briggs KK, Philippon MJ. Relationship between offset angle alpha and hip chondral injury in femoroacetabular impingement. *Arthroscopy.* 2008;24:669-675.
10. Philippon MJ, Briggs KK, Yen YM, Kuppersmith DA. Outcomes following hip arthroscopy for femoroacetabular impingement with associated chondrolabral dysfunction: minimum two-year follow-up. *J Bone Joint Surg Br.* 2009;91:16-23.
11. Philippon MJ, Schenker ML. Arthroscopy for the treatment of femoroacetabular impingement in the athlete. *Clin Sports Med.* 2006;25:299-308.
12. Drehmann F. Drehmann's sign: a clinical examination method in epiphysiolysis (slipping of the upper femoral epiphysis)—description of signs, aetiopathogenetic considerations, clinical experience [in German]. *Z Orthop Ihre Grenzgeb.* 1979;117: 333-344.
13. Tannast M, Siebenrock KA, Anderson SE. Femoroacetabular impingement: radiographic diagnosis—what the radiologist should know. *AJR Am J Roentgenol.* 2007;188:1540-1552.
14. Shindle MK, Voos JE, Nho SJ, et al. Arthroscopic management of labral tears in the hip. *J Bone Joint Surg Am.* 2008;90:2-19.
15. Philippon MJ, Maxwell RB, Johnston TL, et al. Clinical presentation of femoroacetabular impingement. *Knee Surg Sports Traumatol Arthrosc.* 2007;15:1041-1047.
16. Philippon MJ, Souza BGS. Identifying labral tears in daily practice. *Sports Med Update.* 2009;2:3-6.
17. Burnett RS, Della Rocca GJ, Prather H, et al. Clinical presentation of patients with tears of the acetabular labrum. *J Bone Joint Surg Am.* 2006;88:1448-1457.

18. McCarthy JC, Noble PC, Schuck MR, et al. The Otto E. Aufranc Award: The role of labral lesions to development of early degenerative hip disease. *Clin Orthop Relat Res.* 2001;(393):25-37.
19. Maheshwari AV, Malik A, Dorr LD. Impingement of the native hip joint. *J Bone Joint Surg Am.* 2007;89:2508-2518.
20. Murphy SB, Ganz R, Müller ME. The prognosis in untreated dysplasia of the hip. *J Bone Joint Surg Am.* 1995;77:985-989.
21. Heyman CH, Herndon CH. Legg-Perthes disease: a method for the measurement of the roentgenographic result. *J Bone Joint Surg Am.* 1950;32:767-778.
22. Leunig M, Beck M, Kalhor M, et al. Fibrocystic changes at anterosuperior femoral neck: prevalence in hips with femoroacetabular impingement. *Radiology.* 2005;236:237-246.
23. Li PLS, Ganz R. Morphologic features of congenital acetabular dysplasia. *Clin Orthop Relat Res.* 2003;(416):245-253.
24. Kalberer F, Sierra RJ, Madan SS, et al. Ischial spine projection into the pelvis: a new sign for acetabular retroversion. *Clin Orthop Relat Res.* 2008;(466):677-683.
25. Yamamoto Y, Tonotsuka H, Ueda T, Hamada Y. Usefulness of radial contrast-enhanced computed tomography for the diagnosis of acetabular labrum injury. *Arthroscopy.* 2007;232:1290-1294.
26. Fadul DA, Carrino JA. Imaging of femoroacetabular impingement. *J Bone Joint Surg Am.* 2009;91:138-143.
27. Byrd JW. Hip arthroscopy in the supine position. *Oper Tech Sports Med.* 10:184-195, 2002.
28. Glick JM, Sampson TG, Gordon RB, et al. Hip arthroscopy by the lateral approach. *Arthroscopy.* 1987;3:4-12.
29. Kelly BT, Williams RJ 3rd, Philippon MJ. Hip arthroscopy: current indications, treatment options, and management issues. *Am J Sports Med.* 2003;31:1020-1037.
30. Philippon MJ, Stubbs AJ, Schenker ML, et al. Arthroscopic management of femoroacetabular impingement: osteoplasty technique and literature review. *Am J Sports Med.* 2007;35:1571-1580.
31. Philippon MJ,. Schenker ML. A new method for acetabular rim trimming and labral repair. *Clin Sports Med .* 2006;25:293-297.
32. Ilizaliturri VM Jr, Byrd JW, Sampson TG, et al. A geographic zone method to describe intra-articular pathology in hip arthroscopy: cadaveric study and preliminary report. *Arthroscopy.* 2008;24:534-539.
33. Dvorak M, Duncan CP, Day B. Arthroscopic anatomy of the hip. *Arthroscopy.* 1990;6:264-273.
34. Kelly BT, Weiland DE, Schenker M, et al. Arthroscopic labral repair in the hip: surgical technique and review of the literature. *Arthroscopy.* 2005;21:1496-1504.
35. Zumstein M, Hahn F, Sukthankar A, et al. How accurately can the acetabular rim be trimmed in hip arthroscopy. for pincer-type femoral acetabular impingement: a cadaveric investigation. *Arthroscopy.* 2009;25:164-168.
36. Seldes RM, Tan V, Hunt J, et al. Anatomy, histologic features and vascularity of the adult acetabular labrum. *Clin Orthop Relat Res.* 2001;382:232-240.
37. Tan V, Seldes RM, Katz MA, et al. Contribution of acetabular labrum to articulating surface area and femoral head coverage in adult hip joints: an anatomic study in cadavera. *Am J Orthop.* 2001;30):809-812.
38. Ferguson SJ, Bryant JT, Ganz R, et al. An in vitro investigation of the acetabular labral seal in hip joint mechanics. *J Biomech.* 2003;36:171-178.
39. Lavigne M, Parvizi J, Beck M, et al. Anterior femoroacetabular impingement Part 1: techniques of joint-preserving surgery. *Clin Orthop Relat Res.* 2004;(418):61-66.
40. Tannast M, Goricki D, Beck M, et al. Hip damage occurs at the zone of femoroacetabular impingement. *Clin Orthop Relat Res.* 2008;(466):273-280.
41. Ilizaturri VM Jr. Complications of arthroscopic femoroacetabular impingement treatment: a review. *Clin Orthop Relat Res.* 2009;(467):760-768.
42. Philippon MJ, Wolff AB, Briggs KK, et al. Rim reduction for the treatment of pincer-type FAI correlates with pre- and postoperative CE angle. Paper presented at: 2009. Annual Meeting of the American Academy of Orthopaedic Surgeons; February 2009; Las Vegas.
43. Espinosa N, Rothenfluh DA, Beck M, et al. Treatment of femoroacetabular impingement: preliminary results of labral refixation. *J Bone Joint Surg Am.* 2006;88:925-935.
44. Philippon MJ, Arnoczky SP, Torrie A. Arthroscopic repair of the acetabular labrum: a histologic assessment of healing in an ovine model. *Arthroscopy.* 2007;23:376-380.
45. Sampson TG. Arthroscopic treatment of femoroacetabular impingement. *Am J Orthop.* 2008;37:608-612.
46. Philippon MJ, Christensen JC, Wahoff MS. Rehabilitation after arthroscopic repair of intra-articular disorders of the hip in a professional football athlete. *J Sport Rehabil.* 2009;18:118-134.
47. Philippon MJ, Schenker ML, Briggs KK, Maxwell RB. Can microfracture produce repair tissue in acetabular chondral defects? *Arthroscopy.* 2008;24:46-50.
48. Wenger DE, Kendell KR, Miner MR, Trousdale RT. Acetabular labral tears rarely occur in the absence of bony abnormalities. *Clin Orthop Relat Res.* 2004;(426):145-150.
49. Ranawat AS, McClincy M, Sekiya JK. Anterior dislocation of the hip after arthroscopy in a patient with capsular laxity of the hip: a case report. *J Bone Joint Surg Am.* 2009;91:192-197.
50. Enseki KR, Martin RL, Draovitch P, et al. The hip joint: arthroscopic procedures and postoperative rehabilitation. *J Orthop Sports Phys Ther.* 2006;36:516-525.

# CHAPTER 6

# Miscellaneous Problems: Synovitis, Degenerative Joint Disease, and Tumors

Thomas G. Sampson

## GENERAL CONSIDERATIONS

### Synovitis

Synovitis of the hip has many causes. In this chapter, we will discuss only five of the pathologic entities causing primary synovitis—rheumatoid arthritis (RA), calcium pyrophosphate dihydrate crystal deposition disease (CPPD), fatty deposition disease (hyperlipoproteinemia), hemachromatosis, and pyarthrosis—and their arthroscopic treatment.

The role of arthroscopic synovectomy in treating synovial diseases was apparent to the earliest arthroscopists. In almost all pathology of the hip, synovitis is present. Our group has had several undiagnosed cases of hip pain with effusions that were shown to be seronegative rheumatoid arthritis with synovial biopsy. In 1988, Ide and colleagues[1] performed arthroscopic synovectomy for RA on six hips in three patients using mechanical shavers through a two-portal technique, with good results. With the advent of laser and radiofrequency (RF) ablation, there are now three modalities used to débride the synovium. It remains difficult to reach 100% of the joint but with newer, more effective medical management, debulking of the diseased synovium seems to be adequate.

CPPD has not been reported as frequently in the hip as it has in the ligamentum flavum and in the knee, associated with RA.[2,3] Our group has performed synovectomy on two patients for CPPD associated with femoroacetabular impingement. Clearly, it is an entity that should be considered in the differential diagnosis of patients with refractory synovitis.

There are no reports in the arthroscopic literature on the treatment of hyperlipoproteinemia, hemachromatosis, or any of the metabolic arthropathies. Our group has performed partial synovectomy in a few patients thought to have fatty deposition and in one patient with hemachromatosis associated with arthritis. It is presented here only to make the arthroscopic surgeon aware that metabolic arthropathies exist.[4] Metabolic arthropathy appears as white or yellowish plaques on the articular cartilage associated with a mild synovitic reaction. The plaque cannot be removed without destroying the articular cartilage and therefore should be treated with synovectomy only.

Arthroscopic débridement and lavage has become the treatment of choice for septic arthritis in children, adolescents, and adults. This modality has been associated with minimal morbidity and an excellent cure rate.[5-8] McCarthy and associates[9] have reported on successful treatment of septic total hips in two patients using arthroscopic débridement, lavage, and intravenous antibiotics Our group has successfully treated four patients with late hematogenous infections of their total hips arthroscopically. No recurrence has been noted, with the longest follow-up being 20 years, when one patient died from natural causes at the age of 93 years (Fig. 6-1).

### Degenerative Joint Disease

The arthroscopic treatment of degenerative joint disease (DJD) of the hip remains controversial and most challenging and difficult. Even the most experienced hip arthroscopists avoid the procedure in DJD because there are few benchmarks to predict a successful outcome. Prior to 2001, DJD was treated with arthroscopic débridement, labrectomy, synovectomy, and abrasion chondroplasty. In 28 of 290 patients who had partial labrectomies in the presence of DJD, only 21% had a good result compared with a 71% good result rate in those without DJD.[10] Subsequently, with the recognition of femoroacetabular impingement (FAI) and the added correction of the abnormal

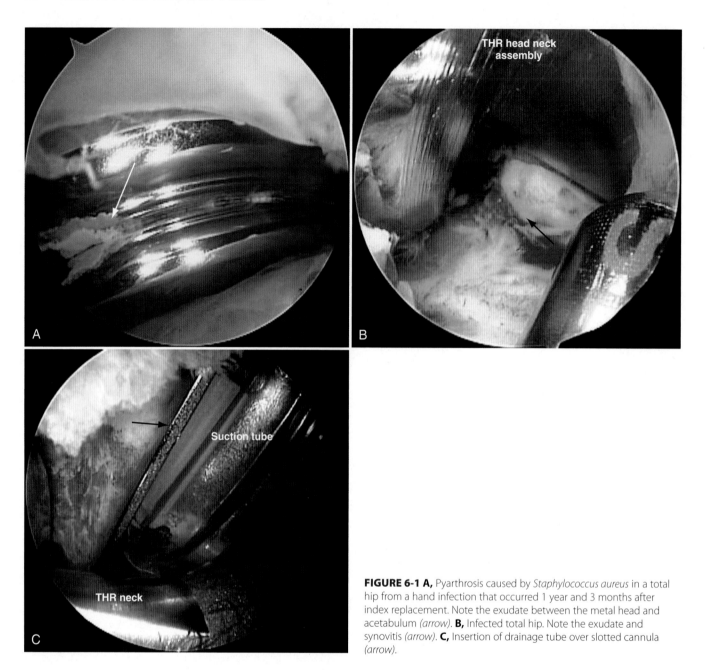

**FIGURE 6-1 A,** Pyarthrosis caused by *Staphylococcus aureus* in a total hip from a hand infection that occurred 1 year and 3 months after index replacement. Note the exudate between the metal head and acetabulum *(arrow).* **B,** Infected total hip. Note the exudate and synovitis *(arrow).* **C,** Insertion of drainage tube over slotted cannula *(arrow).*

morphology, the modified Harris hip score improved significantly from 72 to 92 with an average 4-year follow-up.[11-13]

A residual head-neck deformity from femoral neck fractures has been a cause of FAI and DJD. Reshaping of the deformity has been done using an open surgical dislocation by Eijer and coworkers.[14] Our group has treated the DJD and deformity with an arthroscopic head-neck osteoplasty and débridement, synovectomy, and abrasion chondroplasty with microfracture in three patients.

## Tumors

Essentially all tumors that are amenable to arthroscopic treatment are benign. Pigmented villonodular synovitis (PVNS) and synovial chondromatosis may be considered synovial diseases instead of tumors, and are both difficult to eradicate unless a complete synovectomy can be performed. Frequent recurrences are seen, from inadequate removal of the tumors or inadequate synovectomy.[15-17] Capsulotomy is recommended to expose all areas and recesses of the central and peripheral compartments to remove the loose and attached bodies and ablate the synovium, particularly where the lesions are forming.

Arthroscopic removal of osteoid osteoma of the hip has been described by Glick and colleagues[18] in two cases in the central compartment. Our group has since removed an old, yet active osteoid osteoma from the head-neck junction associated with a cam impingement requiring excision, synovectomy, and head neck osteoplasty (Fig. 6-2).

Heterotopic bone should be considered a pseudotumor of the hip and is most often a complication of trauma or hip

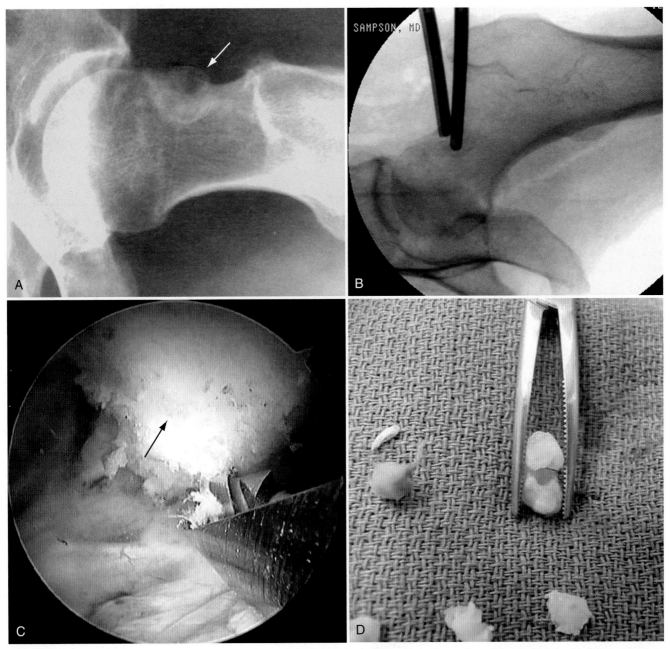

**FIGURE 6-2 A,** Radiograph of a 43-year-old woman with a 10-year history of a painful osteoid osteoma *(arrow).* **B,** Localization with fluoroscopy at surgery. **C,** The mass effect of the osteoid osteoma seen at arthroscopy *(arrow).* **D,** Removed osteoid osteoma, along with multiple loose bodies.

surgery. There are no reports of its treatment using arthroscopic techniques; however, our group favors arthroscopic excision and follow surgery with a single dose of 700 rad of radiation or a strong dose of nonsteroidal anti-inflammatory drugs (NSAIDs) for 3 to 6 weeks. The recurrence rate is lower with the subsequent radiation.

## ANATOMY AND PHYSICAL EXAMINATION

Synovitis of the hip may present with pain in the groin, buttock, and trochanter. The hallmarks of the presentation and examination are associated with an irritable hip. Much like an acute abdomen that is stiff and exquisitely painful on palpation and jarring, the irritable hip is very painful on palpation and rotational movements. Synovitic hips will have pain with all ranges of motion or at the extremes of motion when tested passively. Septic hips may vary as to the level of pain, depending on the organism type and the tenseness of the effusion.

Degenerative joint disease presents with or without a limp, and difficulty walking, sitting, and putting on shoes and socks because of restricted range of motion. With the loss of articular cartilage, a straight leg raise with the knee extended may cause pain in the groin because of the compressive forces of the opposing chondromalacic surfaces of the head and acetabulum. There may be popping and catching with rotation. Loss of internal rotation is almost always present. The Trendelenburg sign and test may be negative in milder cases. Our group has found that if there is at least 50% range of rotational movement when tested passively compared with the normal contralateral side, and if more than 50% of articular cartilage thickness on the anteroposterior (AP) x-ray is present, results show a more than 80% chance of significant improvement that continues for more than 2 years (Fig. 6-3).

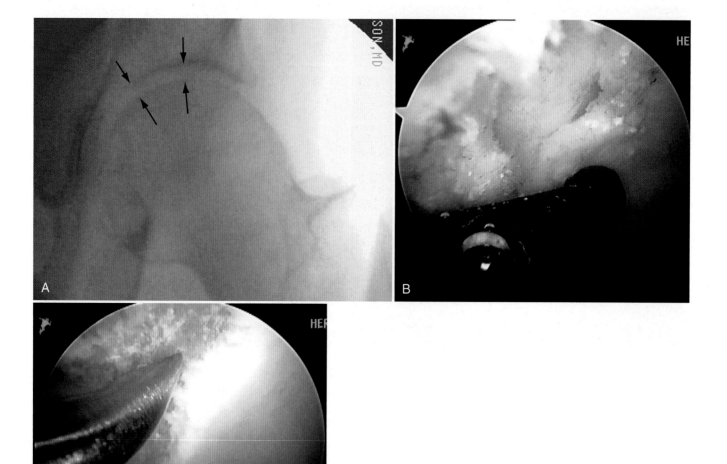

**FIGURE 6-3 A,** Fluororadiograph of a 55-year-old man with 3 years of left hip pain, DJD, and FAI. Note maintenance of the joint space *(arrows)*. After arthroscopic synovectomy, débridement, microfracture, and removal of the cam bump, his modified Harris hip score was still 100 at 5 years postoperatively. **B,** Arthroscopic view of the fragmented acetabular articular cartilage being débrided by an RF probe. **C,** Microfracture of the exposed acetabular bone.

Tumors present with pain and, in many cases, popping and catching. There may be a limp if there is an effusion. Range of motion may be restricted if catching or locking is present. Most patients may present with entirely normal movement. Osteoid osteomas usually cause night pain that is relieved by aspirin or other NSAIDs.[18,19]

## PREOPERATIVE IMAGING AND PLANNING

Routine radiographs are mandatory for preliminary imaging of the hip in all cases of hip symptoms. This should include an AP view of the pelvis, including both hips from the top of the iliac crest to below the lesser trochanters and frog-leg and cross-table lateral views. On the AP view, the tip of the coccyx should be 1 to 2 cm from the pubic symphysis to eliminate pelvic tilt. Magnetic resonance imaging (MRI) and magnetic resonance arthrography (MRA) with gadolinium should be done as an adjunct to the x-rays if clinically indicated.

The findings of synovitis on x-ray may be normal in the early stages may include subtle erosions and cyst formation. On MRI, the findings in RA may include subchondral erosions and hypertrophic synovium.[20] DJD is easily detectable x-rays and MRI scans, with osteophyte formation and joint space narrowing. Because FAI may be the cause in many osteoarthritic hips, a metaplastic bump on the head-neck junction and a rim overgrowth or prominence may be seen. In many cases, a fibro-osseous cyst of varying size appears on the neck, typically within the bump. The MRI shows capsular thickening, chondral erosions, and usually some cysts.

Pigmented villonodular synovitis may only be detected by MRI in the early stages and in late stages with periarticular erosion, effusion, and MR characteristics of hemosiderin deposition in the synovium. In these cases, it is important to examine the entire hip thoroughly, including the peripheral compartment, to ensure as thorough a resection as possible.

Synovial chondromatosis presents as cartilage type or osteocartilage type, with the latter visualized on plain radiographs. MRI images may range from loose bodies from small uniform-sized areas attached to the synovium to large, detached multiple bodies. In some cases, large aggregates and masses are also noted.

In all cases, radiography and MRI identify the diagnosis and location(s) of the lesions to be addressed arthroscopically. The standard techniques of hip arthroscopy are used to confirm the diagnosis. The use of a wide capsulotomy to expose the lesions is recommended. This allows for easier access of the instruments and facilitated removal of masses and loose bodies. The capsulotomy may be done from the central compartment by connecting the portals with an arthroscopic knife, or by an extracapsular method (see later). All peripheral compartment surgery may be done without distraction.

## TECHNIQUE

### Anesthesia Considerations

Most hip arthroscopy is done in an outpatient setting. It is difficult to predict the operative time in many of these cases, especially those with DJD and loose bodies from synovial chondromatosis. Our group performs the procedure with the patient in the lateral decubitus position. Awake patients under regional anesthesia may become uncomfortable lying on their side for the duration of the procedure. For this reason, as well as for relaxation and the need for paralysis, a general anesthetic is recommended.

### Positioning

The supine or lateral position may be used to treat these conditions. The preference and skill of the hip arthroscopist will determine which to use. There are multiple series documenting good outcomes with both techniques.

### Portals

In most arthroscopic procedures for the treatment for synovitis, DJD, and tumors, the standard three portals (anterior, anterolateral, and posterolateral) are used. When more peripheral areas need to be reached, the addition of an anterior and distal portal between 5 and 8 cm from the anterior portal is useful.

### Procedure

The patient is placed in the supine or lateral decubitus position and the appropriate distractor is applied to the affected leg. A C-arm fluoroscope is brought in and, before prepping the patient, a series of four views is taken and recorded. These include AP views in neutral, internal, and external rotation as well as an AP 90-degree view to show the shape and interaction between the head-neck junction and the acetabulum, and to appreciate any loose bodies and their change in position.

Under fluoroscopic control, the long needle is placed through the anterolateral portal directed toward the capsular area at the head-neck junction. There should be about 1 cm of clearance with the greater trochanter. A Nitinol wire is placed through the needle and the skin is incised with a no. 11 blade. The arthroscope trocar sheath assembly is pushed over the wire and the sheath is used to sweep the muscle away from the capsule. The procedure is begun with a 30-degree arthroscope. The pump is started at 50 mm Hg pressure on low flow, allowing a view of the fat pad over the anterior hip capsule. The anterior portal is established with the same technique and a 4-mm switching stick is used to sweep the capsule and palpate the reflected head of the rectus femoris. The key to this approach is identifying the rectus femoris, because the capsule directly beneath covers the anterolateral portion of the labrum (Fig. 6-4).

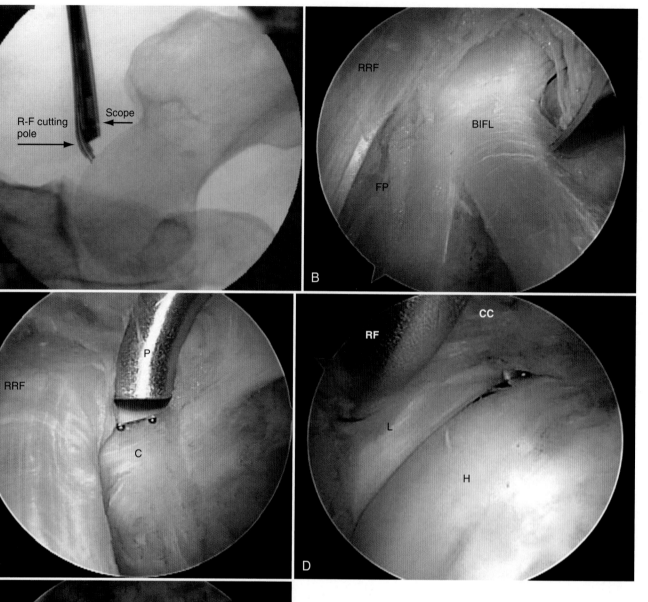

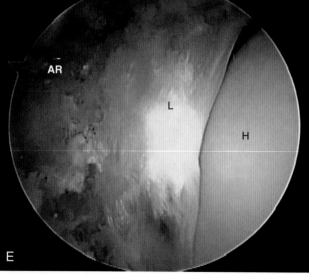

**FIGURE 6-4 A,** C-arm fluoroscopic view of the arthroscope and RF probe over the anterolateral capsule of a left hip before capsulotomy. **B,** Arthroscopic view external to the left anterolateral hip capsule. Note the reflected head of the rectus femoris (RRF), fat pad over the capsule (FP), and band of the iliofemoral ligament (BIFL). **C,** Arthroscopic view external to the left anterolateral hip capsule with the RF probe in place that matches the fluoroscopic view in **A** before capsulotomy. Note the RRF, capsule (C), and RF probe (P). **D,** Arthroscopic view of the cut capsule (CC), with the RF probe retracting the capsule before incising it over the labrum (L). Note the femoral head (H). **E,** Arthroscopic view of the completed capsulotomy exposing the femoral head (H), labrum (L), and acetabular rim (AR), much like what is seen in an arthrotomy.    *Continued*

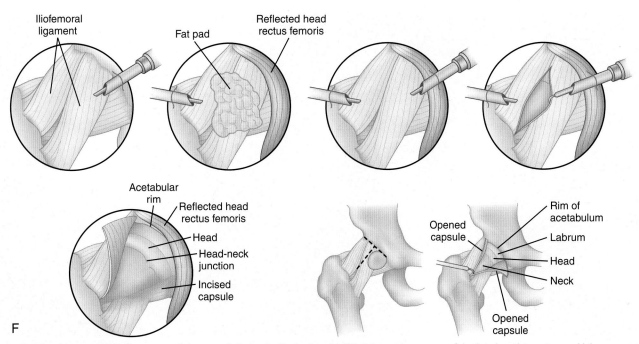

**FIGURE 6-4, cont'd F,** Illustration of the capsule being incised using the RF probe and exposure of the head-neck junction and labrum.

A 4-mm shaver is introduced and the fat is removed to expose the capsule. The capsulotomy is done with an RF probe, beginning at the base of the neck, toward the labrum. Capsular thickening is common and, in my experience, may vary from 2 or 3 mm to 2 cm. By lifting the capsule with the probe before cutting when near the articular cartilage and labrum, exposure may be done without damaging those structures. The capsulotomy is carried up and over the labrum and along the anterior and lateral acetabular rim, between the labrum and the bone.

Synovitis, loose bodies, degenerative tissue, and normal and abnormal anatomy of the head-neck region are visualized similar to an open procedure with the addition of magnification (Fig. 6-5).

Once the peripheral pathology has been identified, the hip is then distracted to enter the central compartment. It may be necessary to create a posterolateral portal to work in all areas of the central compartment. The central compartment is then inspected for pathology methodically, first through the anterolateral portal using a probe from the anterior or posterolateral portal. Moving the scope to the other portals is necessary for complete assessment of the joint.

If loose bodies are present, they are removed with a shaver and graspers. Occasionally, the fat pad hides notch bodies or is fibrotic, and is removed with the shaver. If the notch is filled with a mat of chondromata, the mass is removed with a combination of curettes, picks, and shavers (Fig. 6-6). If the notch has encroaching osteophytes, osteophytectomy using a long 4-mm hip burr, curettes, and picks is preferable to restore the contact forces between the head and acetabular cartilage (Fig. 6-7).[21]

The rim of the acetabulum may have an anterolateral osteophytic ridge. The osteophyte is exposed behind the labrum and removed with a 4-mm hip burr. If cysts are encountered, they are curetted and saucerized with the burr (Fig. 6-8).

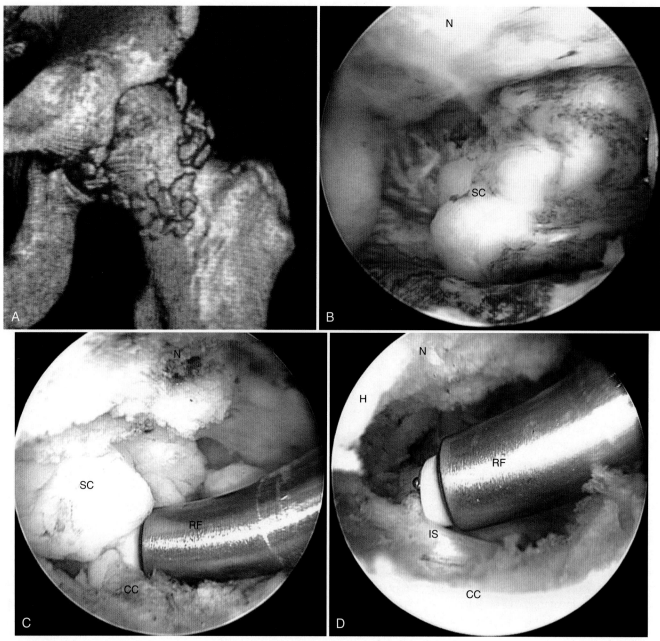

**FIGURE 6-5 A,** Three-dimensional CT scan of the left hip with synovial chondromatosis. **B,** Arthroscopic view of a clump of synovial chondromata (SC) anterior to the femoral neck (N). **C,** Arthroscopic view of a clump of SC anterior to the femoral neck (N) being freed up before extraction with an RF probe (RF). Note the cut capsule (CC). **D,** Arthroscopic view anterior to N in which the mass has been removed, exposing the iliopsoas (IS); the RF is being used to do a synovectomy. Note the femoral head (H).

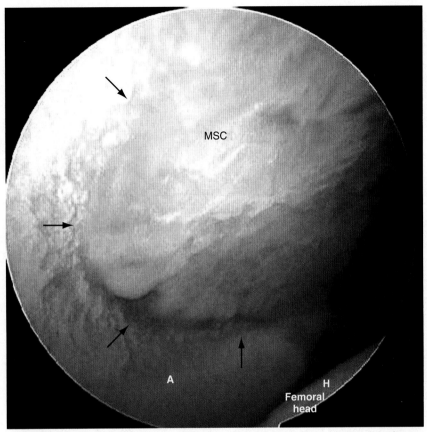

**FIGURE 6-6** View of matted mass of synovial chondromata (MSC) filling the acetabular fossa. Note the acetabulum (A) and femoral head (H).

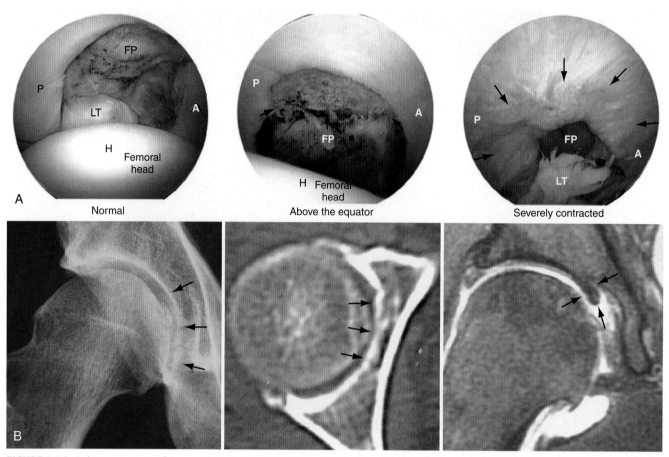

**FIGURE 6-7 A,** Arthroscopic views of the acetabular fossa from normal to arthritic. Note the head (H), ligamentum teres (LT), fat pad (FP), and anterior (A) and posterior (P) views. **B,** AP radiograph (A) of the fossa osteophyte, and CT (B) and MRI (C) scans. Note the notch osteophyte *(arrows).*

*Continued*

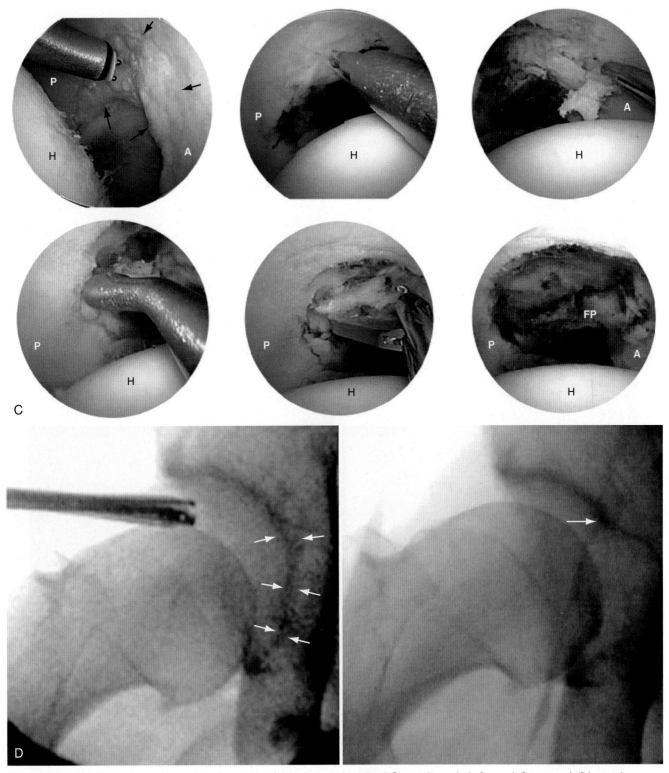

**FIGURE 6-7, cont'd C,** Arthroscopic procedure for excision of a notch osteophyte. **D,** AP fluororadiographs before and after removal of the notch osteophyte *(arrows)*.

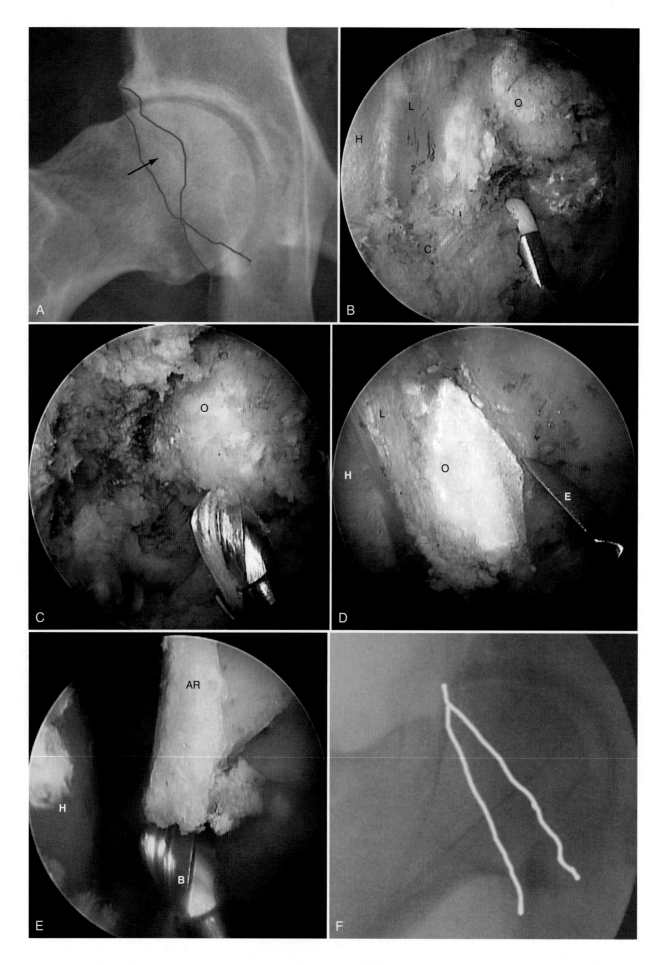

**FIGURE 6-8 A,** AP radiograph in a 46-year-old man with painful DJD. The right hip shows a large, multishaped anterior impingement osteophyte *(arrow)*. **B,** Arthroscopic view of the multishaped anterior rim osteophyte (O), with the soft tissue being dissected away by the RF wand. Note the head (H), labrum (L) and capsule (C). **C,** Arthroscopic view of the osteophyte (O) being excised by the 5-mm burr (B). **D,** Arthroscopic view of an elevator (E) separating the remaining osteophyte (O) away from the rim. **E,** Arthroscopic view of acetabular rim (AR) trimming with the 5-mm burr (B). **F,** Postoperative fluororadiograph showing the correction and removal of the anterior rim osteophyte.

Labral degeneration, tears, or destruction by synovitis are treated with partial labrectomy with the shaver and/or an RF wand. In some cases, a labral repair or refixation is done by abrading the base of the anticipated acetabular attachment with a 4-mm burr, followed by drilling for the anchor of choice, and finally inserting the anchor. The suture is wrapped around the labrum or sewn through with a suture passer or suture relay technique. Finally, the labrum is tied down securing it. It is preferable to place anchors 1 cm apart, which will determine the number of anchors used.

Erosions of the articular cartilage of the head and acetabulum require excision of the delaminated tissue to stable cartilage with a shaver or curette, abrasion and removal of the calcific layer, and microfracture using the awls. Most areas can be reached on the acetabular surface except for zone 6, near the transverse ligament; however, on the femoral head, there is difficulty applying instruments to zones 2m, 3m, 4m, and 6.[22]

In the peripheral compartment, the capsulotomy makes it much easier to find and remove loose bodies. The search should be performed circumferentially around the head and neck, beneath the lateral and medial synovial folds, near the transverse ligament and the distal capsular reflection near the lesser trochanter. Once the loose bodies or PVNS lesions have been removed, a synovectomy using 4-mm straight and curved shavers and RF wands is recommended. A flexible wand may be needed to reach all the areas. By doing as complete a synovectomy as possible, the recurrence rate of the disease will be reduced.

Finally, in the case of DJD, the femoral head-neck junction may need to be reshaped in the same way as with FAI. The neck may have barnacle-like osteophytes that are removed with a shaver, burr, and curettes.

If the hip is arthritic and stiff, a generous capsulectomy is done with the 5-mm shaver, arthroscopic knife, and/or RF probe. In all other situations, the capsule is left open, because it will heal in most cases (Fig. 6-9).

The treatment of septic arthritis involves entering the central compartment first with distraction through an anterolateral portal and placing a shaver through the posterolateral portal to carry out débridement, lavage, and a synovectomy. The peripheral compartment may be reached by releasing traction and flexing the hip to create the space, or by the method of capsulotomy described earlier. Lavaging the hip with more than 3 L of saline is recommended. Drains are placed through a slotted cannula and sewn into the skin. Broad-spectrum intravenous antibiotics are started after adequate cultures are taken. The antibiotic is later changed, based on the results of culture and sensitivity testing. Consideration should always be given to the involvement of an infectious disease consultant.

> **PEARLS & PITFALLS**
>
> - Whether to enter the central compartment first or do a capsulotomy is determined by the preoperative plan and distractibility of the hip. It is preferable to perform a capsulotomy first because most of the work is done in the peripheral compartment and no distraction is needed.
> - Once done with the central compartment, distraction should be released. This avoids unnecessary traction and complication.
> - Repairing the capsule, leaving the capsule open, or performing a capsulectomy should be considered. If the patient has hypermobile joints or there is concern about instability, the capsule is repaired with side to side absorbable no. 1 monofilament suture using suture hooks and retriever graspers.

## POSTOPERATIVE CARE

After wound closure, 30 mL of bupivacaine is administered to all patients. An NSAID such as ibuprofen, celecoxib, or diclofenac is prescribed to reduce the potential for heterotopic bone formation. On the day of surgery, weight bearing on two crutches is begun as tolerated and progressed to one crutch or a cane. When the patient is experiencing little pain on weight bearing, has no sensation of giving way, and has good hip stabilization, use of the crutches or cane can be discontinued. Beginning 1 day after surgery, or when tolerated, the patient is encouraged to ride a stationary bike with little to no resistance for 20 minutes three times daily. The time is increased along with the resistance as tolerated. Sutures are removed at 1 week and elliptical and weight-training exercises are begun, along with distance walking on a treadmill or outside. The patient is taught range of motion exercises and told not to hyperextend for 3 to 6 weeks. At 1 month, the patient is evaluated for symptoms, range of motion, and hip stability. Most patients continue with self-directed advancement of their exercises and activities. If the range of motion is not 80% of normal, physical therapy is advised. Symptoms may continue to some degree, even after successful surgery, for at least 1 year, and patients are advised not to be alarmed if the symptoms fluctuate in intensity and frequency. Most symptoms improve over months. If there is a significant decline, further investigation with a simple x-ray may lead to a diagnosis of failed surgery. Surgical failure in arthritic patients is demonstrated by further loss of joint space or widening of the medial clear space and superior lateral subluxation.

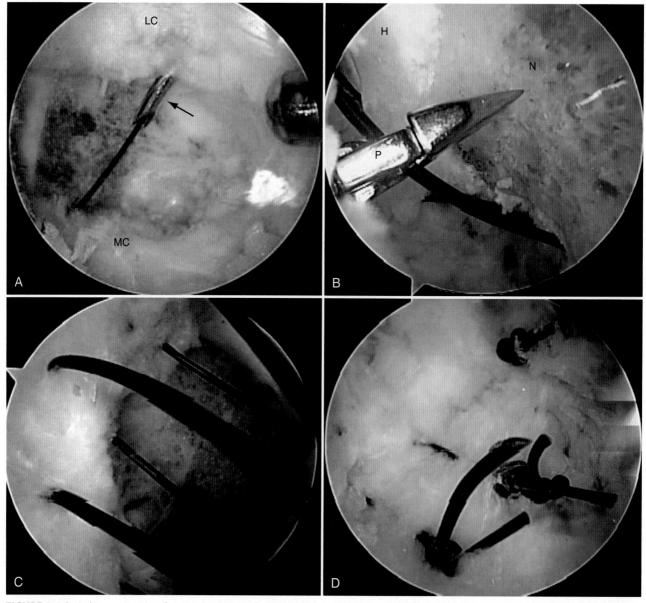

**FIGURE 6-9 A,** Arthroscopic view of a capsular closure of a left hip. The curved suture hook *(arrow)* is shown penetrating the lateral capsule (LC) with a no. 1 absorbable monofilament suture. Note the medial capsule (MC). **B,** Arthroscopic view of a capsular closure of a left hip showing the penetrator (P) grasper grabbing the suture. Note the head (H) and neck (N) of the femur. **C,** Arthroscopic view of a capsular closure of a left hip after a no. 3 suture has been passed before tying. **D,** Arthroscopic view of a capsular closure of a left hip after the sutures have been tied and the capsule closed.

## COMPLICATIONS

Complications may be avoided by paying attention to the length of distraction time and the location of the neurovascular bundles, and taking great care to avoid damage to the articular cartilage.

In our series of 1000 cases, we have found that continuous distraction lasting less than 2 hours results in no sciatic, femoral, or pudendal neuropraxias. We have had five cases of lateral cutaneous neuropraxia; however, all either resolved or the patient accommodated to the patch of numbness on the thigh. Approximately 1% of our cases developed heterotopic bone; in five patients, reoperation was required to alleviate symptoms. There was one nondisplaced femoral neck fracture in a patient treated for DJD and FAI, in which the treatment was placement of a single cannulated screw. This patient has had a final modified Harris hip score of 100 for the last 5 years. We have had no occurrence of deep infections.

## REFERENCES

1. Ide T, Akamatsu N, Nakajima I. Arthroscopic surgery of the hip joint. *Arthroscopy*. 1991;7:204-211.
2. Ishida Y, Oki T, Ono Y, Nogami H. Coffin-Lowry syndrome associated with calcium pyrophosphate crystal deposition in the ligamenta flava. *Clin Orthop Relat Res*. 1992;(275):144-151.
3. Gerster JC, Varisco PA, Kern J, et al. CPPD crystal deposition disease in patients with rheumatoid arthritis. *Clin Rheumatol*. 2006;25:468-469.
4. Timsit MA, Bardin T. Metabolic arthropathies. *Curr Opin Rheumatol*. 1994;6:448-453.
5. Broy SB, Schmid FR. A comparison of medical drainage (needle aspiration) and surgical drainage (arthrotomy or arthroscopy) in the initial treatment of infected joints. *Clin Rheum Dis*. 1986; 12:501-522.
6. Ohl MD, JR Kean, Steensen RN. Arthroscopic treatment of septic arthritic knees in children and adolescents. *Orthop Rev*. 1991;20: 894-896.
7. Blitzer CM. Arthroscopic management of septic arthritis of the hip. *Arthroscopy*. 1993;9:414-416.
8. Kim SJ, Choi NH, Ko SH, et al. Arthroscopic treatment of septic arthritis of the hip. *Clin Orthop Relat Res*. 2003;(407):211-214.
9. McCarthy JC, Jibodh SR, Lee JA. The role of arthroscopy in evaluation of painful hip arthroplasty. *Clin Orthop Relat Res*. 2009;(467):174-180.
10. Farjo LA, Glick JM, Sampson TG. Hip arthroscopy for acetabular labral tears. *Arthroscopy*. 1999;15:132-137.
11. Sampson T. Hip morphology and its relationship to pathology: dyplasia to impingement *Oper Tech Sports Med*. 2005;13:37-45.
12. Sampson T. Arthroscopic treatment of femoroacetabular impingement. *Techniques in Orthopaedics*. 2005;20(1):56-62.
13. Sampson TG. Arthroscopic treatment of femoroacetabular impingement: a proposed technique with clinical experience. *Instr Course Lect*. 2006;55:337-346.
14. Eijer H, Myers SR, Ganz R. Anterior femoroacetabular impingement after femoral neck fractures. *J Orthop Trauma*. 2001;15: 475-481.
15. Boyer T, Dorfmann H. Arthroscopy in primary synovial chondromatosis of the hip: description and outcome of treatment. *J Bone Joint Surg Br*. 2008;90:314-318.
16. Sim FH. Synovial proliferative disorders: role of synovectomy. *Arthroscopy*. 1985;1:198-204.
17. Yamamoto Y, Hamada Y, Ide T, Usui I. Arthroscopic surgery to treat intra-articular type snapping hip. *Arthroscopy*. 2005;21: 1120-1125.
18. Khapchik V, O'Donnell RJ, Glick JM. Arthroscopically assisted excision of osteoid osteoma involving the hip. *Arthroscopy*. 2001; 17:56-61.
19. Alvarez MS, Moneo PR, Palacios JA. Arthroscopic extirpation of an osteoid osteoma of the acetabulum. *Arthroscopy*. 2001;17: 768-771.
20. Sampson T, Bredella M. The hip. In: Stoller DW, ed. *Magnetic Resonance Imaging in Orthopaedics and Sports Medicine*. Philadelphia: Lippincott Williams & Wilkins; 2007:41-304.
21. Daniel M, Iglic A, Kralj-Iglic V. The shape of acetabular cartilage optimizes hip contact stress distribution. *J Anat*. 2005;207: 85-91.
22. Ilizaliturri VM Jr, Byrd JW, Sampson TG, et al., A geographic zone method to describe intra-articular pathology in hip arthroscopy: cadaveric study and preliminary report. *Arthroscopy*. 2008;24:534-539.

## SUGGESTED READINGS

Byrd JWT, *Operative Hip Arthroscopy*. New York: Thieme; 1998: 153-170.

Canale ST, Beaty JH, eds. *Campbell's Operative Orthopaedics, 11th ed.* Vol 1. Philadelphia: Mosby; 2008;736, 855-857, 942.

# Hip Instability

Carlos A. Guanche

Unlike the shoulder, which relies primarily on static and dynamic soft tissue restraints for its stability, the hip depends primarily on its osseous anatomy. The hip's unique soft tissue envelope also plays a role in its stability, particularly when there is any significant deviation from normal.[1] When considering a patient with hip pain that is believed to be at least in some way the result of hip instability, both osseous and soft tissue constraints must be considered. Traumatic dislocation is typically accompanied by a history of an acute event. Atraumatic hip instability can result from repetitive rotational movements. The hypothesized mechanism for this type of instability is a subclinical capsular laxity accompanied by mild hip dysplasia that may progress over time.[2] Generalized laxity and connective tissue disorders are also causes of atraumatic instability.

Treatment of hip instability is largely based on the underlying cause. Diagnosing the cause of the problem begins with a proper history and physical examination, followed by plain radiography. Specialized radiography may be indicated, as well as further imaging. Depending on the diagnosis, treatment may consist of conservative care involving temporary immobilization, activity modification, physical therapy, and eventual return to activity. In refractory cases, surgical capsular repair or labral or capsular treatment may be necessary. In the presence of severe dysplasia or with progression to arthritis, periacetabular osteotomy may be considered. Traumatic dislocations may also require concomitant fragment excision or fixation.

## ANATOMY

Embryologic development is critical to the subsequent development of some forms of instability. Once fused, the acetabular surface is oriented approximately 45 degrees cau-

dally and 15 to 20 degrees anteriorly. Significant alterations in acetabular version or inclination, as well as its orientation relative to the femoral head or neck, can affect the joint capsule and ligaments. The suction effect that relies on joint congruency for its function may also be compromised. The variability of this orientation may be a factor in the development of hip instability and needs to be considered in any treatment algorithm.

Although relying largely on its bony anatomy, hip stability is complemented by the acetabular labrum and capsuloligamentous complex. In the neutral anatomic position, the anterior part of the femoral head is not engaged in the acetabulum. The acetabular labrum compensates for this by covering this portion of the femoral head. The labrum is attached to the transverse acetabular ligament anteriorly and posteriorly at the base of the fovea and proceeds to run around the circumference of the acetabular rim.[1] The labrum deepens the "socket" and aids in maintaining the suction effect that provides additional hip stability. Absence of the labrum can lead to a loss of this suction effect, as well as increased cartilage surface consolidation as a result of the loss of hydration, thereby increasing contact pressures.[3-5] Proprioceptors and nociceptors have been identified within the labrum and may explain the decreased proprioception and increased pain in the athlete with a torn labrum.[6] Much like the meniscus in the knee, the labrum is largely avascular, except for the most peripheral portion near the capsule, limiting its ability to heal.[7]

The labrum is not, however, a stand-alone structure. It functions in conjunction with the capsuloligamentous complex. The fibrous hip capsule and its ligaments are like a thick sleeve. Anteriorly, this complex primarily consists of the iliofemoral ligament (ligament of Bigelow), a 12- to 14-mm thick structure shaped like an inverted Y. It provides resistance to hip extension beyond neutral and resists external rotation. The pubofemoral ligament, which arises from the pubic portion of the acetabular rim and passes below the neck of the femur to blend with the most inferior fibers of the iliofemoral ligament, reinforces the inferior and anterior capsules, resisting extension and abduction. The ischiofemoral ligament reinforces the posterior surface of the capsule and has a spiraling pattern. Finally, the zona orbicularis is a deep layer of fibers within the capsule that forms a circular pattern around the femoral neck, constricting the capsule and helping maintain the femoral head within the acetabulum.[1]

The position of maximum hip joint stability is in full extension because it is in this position that the twisted orientation of the capsular ligaments causes a screw-home effect.[1] However, the articular surfaces of the hip joint are not in optimal contact in this position (the close-packed position). Optimal contact occurs in the loose packed position of flexion and lateral rotation as the ligaments uncoil. The greatest risk of traumatic dislocation, then, is when the joint is between the close-packed and maximally congruent position (flexed and adducted position). The ligamentum teres and psoas tendon are two extra-articular structures about the hip that deserve additional discussion. The ligamentum has no real stabilizing effect on the joint, whereas the psoas protects the anterior intermediate capsule, which is devoid of ligamentous protection.

## CLINICAL EVALUATION

### History

Making the diagnosis of hip instability can be a diagnostic dilemma. Hip instability can manifest as overtly as frank traumatic dislocation or can be as obscure as occult groin pain or clicking. Hip pain, clicking, or "giving way" in the young adult patient may arise from any number of anatomic structures. The picture can be further complicated by referred pain from the lumbosacral region as well as the genitourinary tract and abdominal wall.[8] Age also plays a significant role in determining a differential diagnosis for hip pain.[9] In children, hip dislocation, bony avulsions, apophyseal injuries, fractures, slipped capital femoral epiphysis (SCFE), Legg-Perthes disease, developmental dysplasia of the hip (DDH), and toxic and septic arthritis are all potential causes.[9]

The history should include a qualitative assessment of the main complaint to determine whether it is primarily pain, clicking, catching, or instability. A golfer may describe weakness in the involved leg while swinging for power. Pain may also occur after long periods of sitting, when getting out of a car, or rising from a chair. Timing of the onset of the complaint is also essential. Precipitating factors, as well as potential referred or systemic causes, must be assessed.

## Physical Examination

Antalgic gait patterns in which there is shortening of the stance phase and step length on the affected side can result from instability. A Trendelenburg gait may indicate an attempt to bring the center of gravity over the affected side to decrease the moment arm across that hip joint.[10] The patient with atraumatic instability may be able to demonstrate subluxation or dislocation of the involved hip, although this is rare.

Traumatic hip instability can manifest with pain on prone extension–external rotation of the involved hip. A positive axial distraction test can be confirmed with a positive vacuum sign on dynamic fluoroscopy (Fig. 7-1).[1] Anterior apprehension may also be elicited with the patient in the lateral decubitus position while suspending the affected leg in slight abduction (Fig. 7-2). The presence of a positive examination indicates capsular laxity in traumatic and atraumatic instability.

In some patients, and with proper relaxation, a sense of the end range of capsular tightness and the end point of the ligamentum teres can be obtained by the supine external rotation test, in which the patient is placed supine and the affected leg is suspended in 30 degrees of flexion by the examiner. With gentle external rotation, while the patient is relaxed, the end point of external rotation can be assessed (Fig. 7-3). Also, a comparison can be made with the contralateral (and presumably normal) extremity. If there is a significant increase in external rotation as compared with the normal extremity, laxity of the Y ligament can be inferred. Also, if a large anterior labral tear exists, audible snapping and reproduction of pain can be elicited.

Range of motion of the hip joint is also important to document. Supine external rotation should be measured in the normal and affected extremities. Also, rotation of the flexed hip varies with version of the acetabulum. In excessive anteversion, an excess of internal rotation is noted.

## IMAGING

Imaging should always begin with plain radiographs. The standard views are a standing anteroposterior (AP) pelvic view, as well as AP and lateral views of the affected hip. Apart from being able to detect the common radiographic features of trauma, plain radiographs can also help detect femoroacetabular impingement.

Several radiographic indices have been described to differentiate normal from abnormal osseous anatomy based on the AP pelvic radiograph. The Tonnis angle is used to assess lateral subluxation of the femoral head and subsequent increased forces across the weight-bearing acetabulum (Fig. 7-4).[11] A measurement of less than 10 degrees is considered normal.

The center edge angle of Wiberg assesses acetabular inclination (Fig. 7-5). This angle should measure at least 20 to 25 degrees to be considered normal.[12,13] One can estimate acetabular version using the AP pelvis by looking for a crossover sign (Fig. 7-6). The two lines involved estimate the posterior and anterior rims of the acetabulum. The posterior rim

*Text continued on p. 112.*

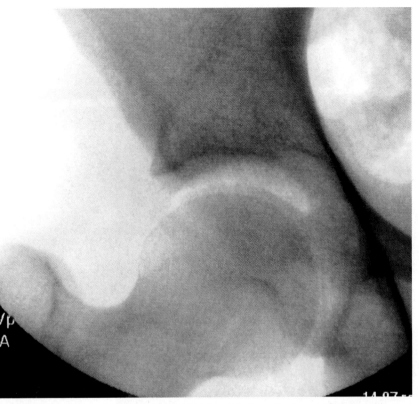

**FIGURE 7-1** Suction seal effect of the joint. This is anintraoperative image of 16-year-old patient with repetitive use instability caused by high-level gymnastics participation. Minor axial traction (15 lb) causes significant distraction and subluxation of the joint.

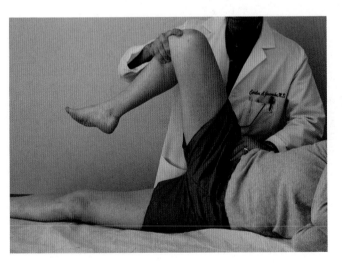

**FIGURE 7-2** Apprehension position. The patient is placed in the lateral decubitus position and the affected extremity is supported by the examiner. The examiner uses the other arm to push the hip in an anterior direction as pressure is applied over the posterior aspect of the greater trochanter. In symptomatic patients, a sensation of subluxation can sometimes be elicited, whereas in others, there is a reproduction of their pain.

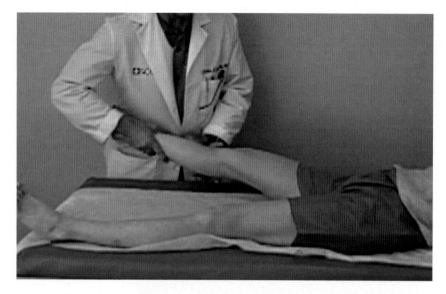

**FIGURE 7-3** Supine external rotation. The patient is in the supine position while the examiner rests the affected extremity in both arms. Gentle maximal external rotation is performed on the leg while the patient attempts to relax. The total external range of motion should be assessed as compared to the contralateral extremity. In addition, a sense of the end point is also obtained.

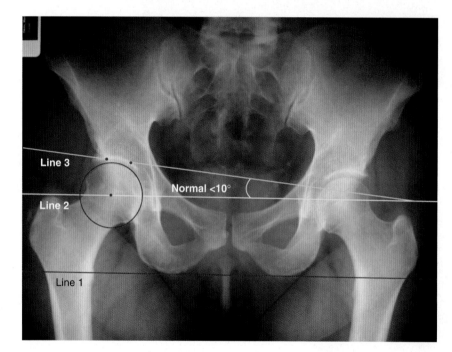

**FIGURE 7-4** AP radiograph showing the technique of measuring the Tonnis angle (normal, <10 degrees). In this case, the *red line* (line 1) connecting the two ischial tuberosities is the reference line on which all other lines are based. The *yellow line* (line 2) is a line drawn parallel to line 1 through the center of the femoral head. The angle formed between line 2 and a third line connecting two points demarcating the sourcil or weight-bearing surface of the acetabulum is the Tonnis angle. *(Adapted from Delaney S, Dussault RG, Kaplan PA, et al. Radiographic measurements of dysplastic adult hips.* Skeletal Radiol. *1997;26:75-81.)*

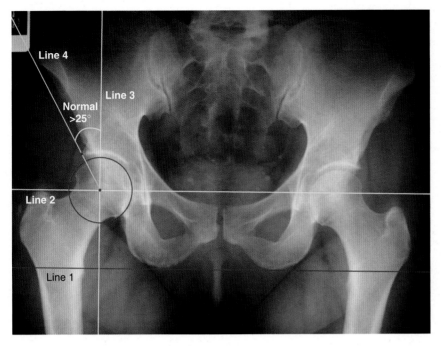

**FIGURE 7-5** AP radiograph showing the measurement technique for the center edge angle of Wiberg. Line 2 is made through the center of the femoral heads. Line 3 is a line directly perpendicular to line 2, and the angle between this line and line 4 (a line from the center of the femoral head to the lateral edge of the acetabulum). This angle should be greater than 25 degrees, with 20 to 25 degrees being considered borderline. *(Adapted from Delaney S, Dussault RG, Kaplan PA, et al. Radiographic measurements of dysplastic adult hips.* Skeletal Radiol. *1997;26:75-81.)*

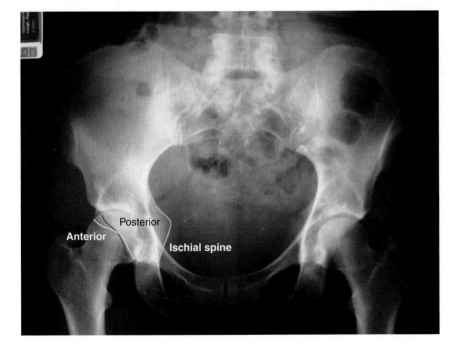

**FIGURE 7-6** AP radiograph demonstrating the crossover sign indicating acetabular retroversion. Note that the *red line* (representing the anterior wall of the acetabulum) crosses the *yellow line* (representing the posterior wall of the acetabulum). Also of note is the visualization of the ischial tuberosity *(blue line)*, which is normally superimposed by the acetabulum, but easily visible in the retroverted acetabulum.

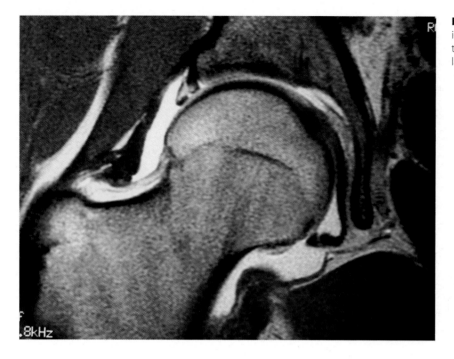

**FIGURE 7-7** MRI scan (T2-weighted coronal image) of a patient with hip instability secondary to excessive capsular volume. Also note the large labral tear that is evident in this image.

is traced from the ischial tuberosity superolaterally to the roof of the acetabulum. The anterior rim is traced from the teardrop in a superior and lateral direction along the rim to the roof. If these lines cross, it is estimated that the acetabulum is retroverted; if not, it is assumed that the acetabular version is within the normal 10- to 15-degree anterior version.[14,15]

When evaluating a patient with potential residual dysplasia, the faux profile view is often used to evaluate anterior and lateral coverage of the femoral head by the acetabulum. Although plain radiographs are sufficient for diagnosis in a number of cases, there are pathologic entities that require further investigation. Imaging of bony lesions about the hip is best accomplished using computed tomography (CT) because it provides the greatest spatial resolution of bony structures. Cases of questionable hip dysplasia should use CT in preoperative planning. The use of intra-articular contrast in CT arthrography can increase the contrast between cartilage and labral tissue.[8]

Magnetic resonance imaging (MRI) has become the most reliable means of diagnosing unresolved hip pathology in addition to direct visualization and is often useful in cases of instability. MRI has been shown to demonstrate inflammatory arthropathies and joint effusions effectively, but has been less accurate in assessing articular cartilage lesions.[8,16,17] Contrast MRI studies in patients with a torn labrum or torn iliofemoral ligament can result in a larger volume of intra-articular contrast, and thus indirectly confirm the diagnosis of instability (Fig. 7-7).[1]

## TREATMENT CONSIDERATIONS

### Atraumatic Instability

As is the case in the shoulder, in which numerous types of instability have been described, the separation between traumatic and atraumatic instability in the hip is often difficult. For the purpose of this chapter, only those instability syndromes that are the direct result of a distinct traumatic event that caused a discrete subluxation or frank dislocation will be considered as traumatic instability. All other congenital dysplasias and connective tissue disorders, as well as repetitive use injuries and idiopathic syndromes, will be considered as atraumatic.

Congenital connective tissue disorders can predispose a patient to atraumatic hip instability. There have been very few reports in the literature of habitual hip dislocation that have not been accompanied by Ehlers-Danlos syndrome, arthrochalasis multiplex congenital, Marfan's syndrome, Down syndrome, or congenital or acquired hip dysplasia.[1] As opposed to frank episodes of subluxation or dislocation that may be seen in atraumatic shoulder instability, idiopathic hip instability often presents with a more subtle pattern. In a review of five cases, a syndrome of idiopathic hip instability was described, in which all patients presented with a long history of snapping in the groin, gait disturbances, and pain in the provocative position of hip flexion, adduction, and internal rotation.[18] Symptoms were alleviated by extension abduction and external rotation (maneuvers analogous to the Barlow and Ortolani signs), thus suggesting a posterior instability. When awake patients had their affected hip subjected to gentle manual traction, 4 to 10 mm of inferior subluxation was seen. The force used to subluxate the hip in these cases was much less than the 400 N of axial force described as necessary to create a radiographic vacuum sign of subluxation.[19] All this evidence led the authors to postulate that subclinical hip dysplasia, combined with capsuloligamentous laxity, causes a break in the suction mechanism of the hip during gait, causing a popping sensation. Presuming that the instability was largely posteriorly directed and that preoperative arthrograms showed posterior capsular redundancy, one patient underwent open posterior capsular plication.

Atraumatic instability has also been attributed to a deficient labrum associated with redundant capsular or ligamentous tissue.[1] This deficient complex can create an abnormal load distribution caused by a transiently incongruent joint. The screw-home mechanism caused by the dynamic nature of the hip capsule and its associated ligaments may help explain why pelvic rotation and external rotation of the hip commonly elicit symptoms of instability. Professional and high-level athletes who participate in sports that require repeated hip rotation (e.g., football, golf, gymnastics) are susceptible to overuse injuries to the labrum and capsuloligamentous complex. Tears of the labrum or iliofemoral ligament can result in insufficiency and cause an increased tension on the joint capsule, which can be further exacerbated in patients with slight superior and lateral inclination of the acetabulum. In addition, cadaveric analysis of hip stability following capsular venting and a 15-mm labral tear has shown that positions of hip extension, when combined with abduction or external rotation, result in large strains in the anterior labrum.[20]

Labral degeneration, combined with subtle rotational hip instability secondary to redundant capsular tissue in elite athletes, has been described. Ten patients were treated with arthroscopic labral débridement and thermal capsulorrhaphy. All patients had improvement in their Harris hip scores, with 83% having significant improvement in their symptoms at 12- to 24-month follow-up.[1] In contrast, Santori and Villar have reported only 67.5% success in 58 cases at a mean 3.5-year follow-up with labral débridement without capsular treatment.[21] Alternatively, plication can also be performed by passing nonabsorbable, braided suture through the capsule, thus imbricating the capsular tissue (Fig. 7-8).[7]

Although subtle hip dysplasia combined with capsular laxity and labral pathology can lead to symptomatic hip instability amenable to arthroscopic treatment, care must be taken to recognize more significant dysplasias. Overtly dysplastic hips typically share common abnormalities that occur to a greater or lesser extent, depending on the severity.[22] The true acetabulum is usually shallow, lateralized, anteverted, and deficient anteriorly and superiorly. There may also be underdevelopment of the entire pelvis. On the femoral side, the femoral head is usually small and the neck is usually excessively anteverted and short, with an increased neck-shaft angle. The greater trochanter may be displaced posteriorly and the femoral canal may be narrow.[23,24] The presence of significant hip dysplasia in the adult can be ascertained using primarily plain radiography.

A patient who presents with radiographic evidence of dysplasia but little or no symptomatology should be treated nonsurgically with strengthening and proprioceptive training of the hip and trunk musculature.[23] Nonsteroidal antiinflammatory drugs (NSAIDs) can be used and combined with cessation of high-impact activities. The patient should be educated about the potential natural history of increasing instability and the potential development of degenerative arthritis.

Surgical intervention should be reserved for those patients who fail conservative management and have persistent symptoms. Arthroscopic treatment in the patient with significant dysplasia is not indicated. In addition, significant labral hypertrophy occurs in these patients. The role of this excess labral tissue has not been completely elucidated, but it may be significant in its effect on joint stability. Aggressive resection of this tissue can accelerate degenerative changes and possibly lead to premature degeneration. Pelvic and

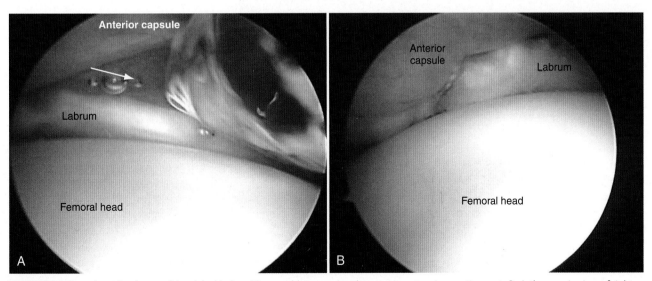

**FIGURE 7-8** Capsular redundancy of the right hip in a 16-year-old gymnast with no major macrotraumatic event. **A,** Arthroscopic view of right hip viewed from the anterolateral portal while in the peripheral compartment. The perilabral sulcus *(arrow)* is seen to be large. The labrum is relatively normal. **B,** View following capsulorrhaphy using suture anchors. Note the obliteration of the perilabral sulcus, with the suture in place immediately proximal to the acetabular rim.

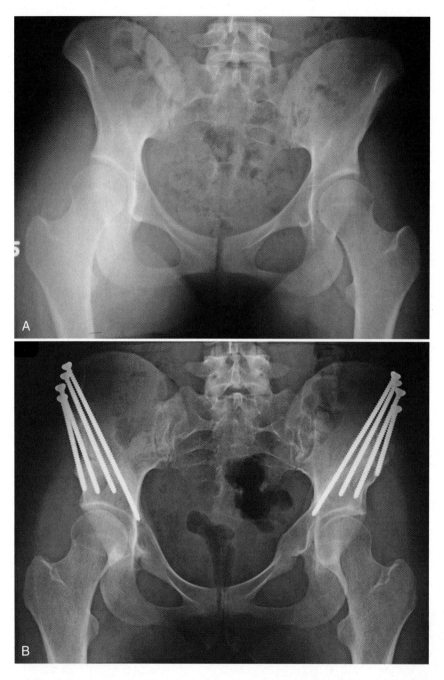

**FIGURE 7-9** Periacetabular osteotomy. **A,** 19-year-old woman with history of hip pain and increasing disability. **B,** Postoperative radiograph following periacetabular osteotomy

femoral osteotomies, arthrodesis, resection arthroplasty, and replacement arthroplasties have all been described as potential treatment options.[23] Osteotomies that may be expected to slow the progression of degenerative changes by distributing weight-bearing forces across the hip joint better have been described. These procedures may also provide better preservation of bone stock for potential subsequent arthroplasty (Fig. 7-9).

## Traumatic Instability

The most common mechanism for hip dislocation is a dashboard motor vehicle injury with a posteriorly directed force against a flexed knee and hip. During athletic activities, dislocations may occur via a forward fall onto a flexed knee with the hip flexed or a blow from behind while down on all four limbs (Fig. 7-10).[25,26] Sports such as American football, skiing, jogging, gymnastics, basketball, biking, and soccer have all had reports of traumatic dislocations (Fig. 7-11).[27-29] Excessive capsular laxity has been associated with these types of dislocations.[30,31] Irrespective of the degree of initial trauma, if normal capsular healing fails to occur, persistent laxity may remain and predispose the patient to instability (Fig. 7-12). Two cases of posterior dislocation following minor trauma while playing soccer have been reported, probably secondary to large posterior capsular redundancy.[32] Similarly, recurrent

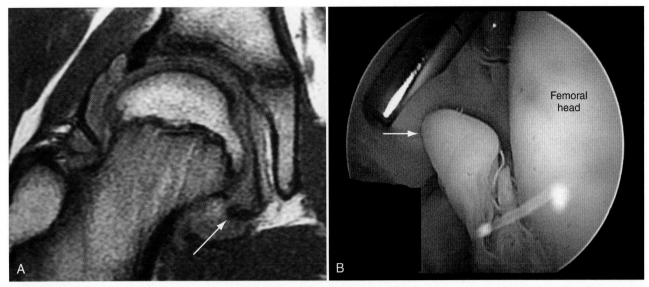

**FIGURE 7-10** Tear of the ligamentum teres following right hip subluxation. **A,** T2-weighted coronal image. The tear is seen at the inferior margin of the acetabulum *(arrow)*. **B,** Arthroscopic view of ligamentum tear *(arrow* points to avulsed end). The view is from the anterolateral portal.

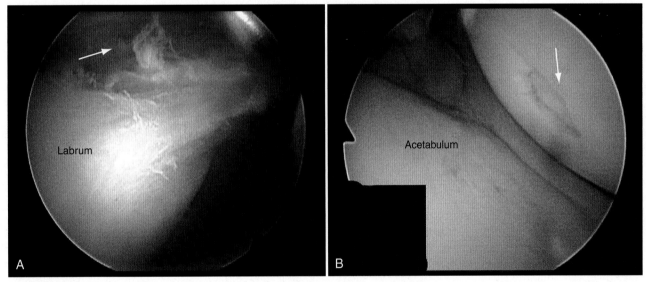

**FIGURE 7-11** Labral tear following dislocation of the right hip in a 19-year-old college basketball player (viewed from the anterolateral portal). **A,** Note the significant synovial reaction *(arrow)* around the labral tearing. **B,** Focal femoral head defect *(arrow)* in the same patient.

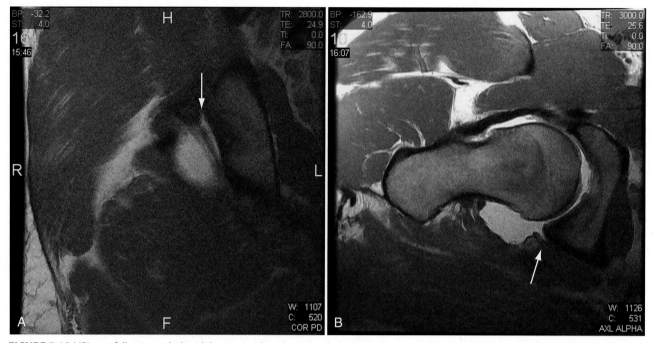

**FIGURE 7-12** MRI scan following right hip dislocation with no bony involvement. **A,** Torn posterior capsule; T1-weighted coronal image through the posterior aspect of the joint. The tear is seen longitudinally at the margin of the posterior labrum *(arrow)*. To the right of the *arrow* is the posterior acetabular wall. **B,** T1-weighted axial image depicting a posterior capsulolabral avulsion *(arrow)*.

anterior dislocations have occurred as a result of excessive anterior capsular redundancy.[33] These patients have been treated nonoperatively with brief immobilization, physical therapy, and activity modification. Open capsular shift or repair has been particularly successful in preventing further dislocation.[34] Arthroscopic treatment of this type of capsular laxity using thermal capsulorrhaphy or capsular plication combined with labral débridement has shown promising early results while potentially avoiding the open surgical complications of heterotopic ossification and osteonecrosis of the femoral head.[1]

Hip arthroscopy has been shown to be an important part of the armamentarium in the effort to at least delay the onset of post-traumatic degenerative joint disease (DJD) following traumatic dislocation.[35,36] Residual intra-articular bony or osteochondral fragments may be responsible for the development of DJD in complex dislocations. The incidence of osteoarthritis secondary to traumatic hip dislocation has been reported between 24% to 57%, depending on the severity of the trauma.[37] Simple dislocations (without radiographic evidence of fracture) have been shown to have the lowest incidence. However, the incidence of post-traumatic DJD in these injuries is still 24%.[38]

Nonconcentric reduction after a traumatic dislocation is considered an absolute indication for operative intervention. The presence of loose bodies (LBs), however, has been considered a relative indication, particularly if the reduction is concentric and the LBs are located below the fovea.[35] An in vivo rabbit model has shown that free cartilaginous loose particles inside the joint increase chondrolytic enzyme activity and induce secondary arthrosis.[39] Because 24% of simple dislocations have been shown to develop subsequent DJD, the literature would support that LBs should be addressed prophylactically, and arthroscopy is an excellent vehicle for accomplishing this (Fig. 7-13).[38]

Mullis and Dahners[36] have reported on a series of 36 patients treated with arthroscopy following dislocation. Excluding procedures in which a repeat arthroscopy was performed for retained LBs, the average time to surgery was 15 days. Of 36 patients, 25 (69%) had radiographic evidence of LBs (nonconcentric reduction and/or radiographically visible LBs). In 9 patients, there was a concentric reduction without radiographic LBs. Intraoperatively, 33 of 36 patients(92%) were found to have LBs. Of the 9 patients with no preoperative radiographic evidence of LBs, 7 (78%) had some found at arthroscopy (Fig. 7-14).

In a 15-year experience with hip arthroscopy after traumatic dislocation, 10 joints in nine patients were treated 1 to 7 days postdislocation.[35] Seven hips were classified as Thompson-Epstein (TE) I injuries, two type II, one type IV, and one central fracture dislocation. All dislocations had arthroscopic lavage and débridement and 7 of 10 joints revealed previously unrecognized loose osteochondral fragments. At a minimum of 5 years follow-up, 8 of 10 joints were asymptomatic. One joint (Pipken type 3 femoral head fracture) went on to develop femoral head AVN that was not symptomatic. The one TE IV injury developed hip joint DJD at 1 year. These results prompted the authors to recommend arthroscopic débridement for all TE types I and II dislocations, but not types III and IV.

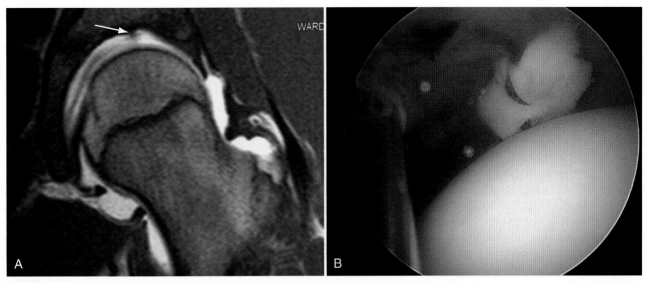

**FIGURE 7-13** Loose cartilaginous bodies in a left hip following dislocation in a collegiate basketball player. **A,** MRI scan (coronal T1-weighted image) reveals a cartilaginous loose body *(arrow)* not evident on plain films. **B,** View from anterior portal. A loose body is silhouetted by synovial tissue.

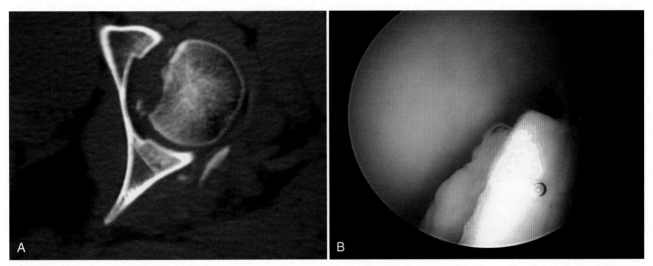

**FIGURE 7-14** Loose bodies in the hip with nonconcentric reduction. **A,** CT scan through the center of the femoral head depicting multiple loose bodies within the joint. **B,** Intraoperative image of loose osteocartilaginous fragment that was removed.

Philippon and colleagues[26] have recently documented acute dislocations in 14 professional athletes. The findings of importance in their study were a significant association between dislocations and additional findings, including significant labral tears (100%), as well as multiple LBs and osteochondral injuries on the acetabular and femoral surfaces in 73% of cases. In addition, 73% had tears of the ligamentum teres. Finally, there were 9 patients (60%) who had evidence of femoroacetabular impingement by radiographic and arthroscopic evaluation.

There has been some concern regarding the timing of arthroscopy after traumatic dislocation in terms of the risk of avascular necrosis (AVN), prompting those concerned to recommend a 6-week waiting period postdislocation before performing arthroscopy. In two of the previously discussed series, however, arthroscopic surgery was performed in the first 2 weeks.[35,36] The only complications observed in the Mullis and Dahners study were three repeat procedures for retained LBs and some fluid extravasation into the gluteal compartment that resolved without incident. Although the possibility of extravasation and subsequent significant complication exists, it can be mitigated by keeping the pressure on the arthroscopic pump low (if one is used). Also, expeditious management of the pathology with limited exposure to inflow of fluid will avoid this issue. In cases in which extended surgical procedures are undertaken, it is important to palpate the abdomen and maintain a watchful eye on the patient's vital signs to note any ongoing extravasation, particularly into the abdominal cavity.[36] Yamamoto and associates[35] had one case of AVN that developed in a patient with a Pipken type 3 injury.

## SURGICAL TECHNIQUE

The standard hip arthroscopy techniques described in other chapters of this text will suffice with respect to positioning. Either the lateral or supine position is effective for dealing with the sequelae of dislocations, such as labral tearing and LBs. One critical element in the procedure includes an examination under anesthesia of both the affected extremity and the presumably normal contralateral hip. The decisions that need to be made refer to laxity of the capsular tissues, and whether there is a radiographic vacuum sign in those with atraumatic instability. Also, the direction of instability and positions of stability need to be documented.

A complete diagnostic examination of the hip joint is also critical and includes the peripheral compartment. There are many cases in which the central compartment diagnostic evaluation reveals only minimal trauma and possibly some chondral abnormalities, without any evident LBs. On entering the peripheral compartment, however, a loose body can be found and may be responsible for some of the mechanical symptoms that the patient is experiencing.

The first technique to discuss with regard to the challenges presented by dislocations is that of labral repair. A variety of techniques are available for repair of labral detachment; these are similar to the experience in the shoulder. The specific challenges presented by the hip include the limited maneuverability within the joint and sometimes the degree of damage to the labrum, precluding a good repair. The specific techniques have been described in the chapter on labral injury (see Chapter 3).

The issue of capsular laxity is of particular interest, especially in patients with atraumatic instability. The amount of laxity that is normal is difficult to quantify and there are no scientific studies to date that offer objective criteria with respect to imbricating the capsule. It has been my experience that those patients who have a significant radiographic vacuum under anesthesia or frankly subluxate with an examination under anesthesia (EUA) are those who warrant a capsular repair.

Once all the labral pathology has been addressed, the amount of capsular redundancy is assessed. It is important to assess the laxity over the area that is presumed to be abnormal based on the EUA and the mechanism of injury, if one is known. Most commonly, the anterior capsule is involved in atraumatic patients. The assessment and treatment of this problem are undertaken from the peripheral compartment with traction removed and the leg in approximately 45 degrees of flexion. To imbricate the capsule, an accessory portal needs to be established, in addition to the standard anterior and anterolateral portals. The portal that is typically established is termed the *midanterolateral* (MAL) *portal* and is established midway between the anterior and anterolateral portals, creating an equilateral triangle between the three portals (Fig. 7-15). This portal is used for manipulation of the sutures between portals.

In the typical case, the imbrication is undertaken in a medial to lateral direction. In patients in whom there is a very large perilabral sulcus, a proximal to distal imbrication is technically simpler easier to accomplish (see Fig. 7-8). When a medial to lateral imbrication is undertaken, the first step is to isolate the capsule on both the intra-articular and extra-articular spaces. The extra-articular preparation is undertaken by pulling the arthroscope out of the capsule (arthroscope in the anterolateral [AL] portal). Once the scope is out of the joint, the anterior portal is used to elevate the soft tissues away from the capsule to visualize the area where the imbrication will take place. Once an area of approximately 2 cm² is cleared, preparation is made for suture passing. The anterior portal serves as the portal for delivery of sutures from outside the joint and the MAL serves as the portal to grasp the sutures within the joint. Using a suture penetrator device, one suture is placed through the capsule and grasped from the AL portal. The other limb of the suture is now passed through the capsule, approximately 1 cm more lateral than the first limb. This limb is retrieved through the AL portal and shuttled outside the cannula. A second suture is now passed proximally or distally to the first, depending on the configuration of the first suture. Once the two sutures are passed, the arthroscope is placed outside the joint again and the sutures are tied (see Fig. 7-8). Confirmation of appropriate tightening of the joint can be obtained by visualization of the joint through the AL portal.

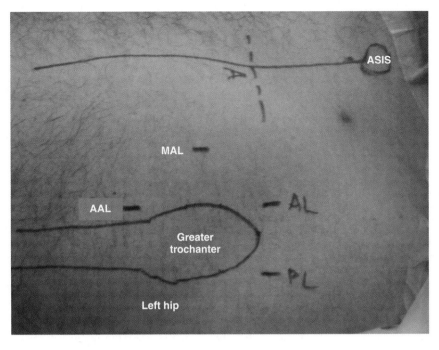

**FIGURE 7-15** This midanterolateral (MAL) portal was established midway between the anterior (A) and anterolateral (AL) portals. An equilateral triangle is formed between the two standard portals and the MAL. AAL, accessory anterolateral; ASIS, anterior-superior iliac spine; PL, posterolateral.

## PEARLS & PITFALLS

- Thoughtful assessment of radiographs

  The most important consideration in any patient with a presumed unstable hip is to determine the degree of bony abnormality. In cases of mild dysplasia, there is certainly a good potential outcome with a properly performed arthroscopic stabilization. In cases of more severe dysplasia, consideration should be given to more complex (and open) procedures, including periacetabular osteotomies.

- Examination under anesthesia

  Examine each patient under anesthesia prior to any instrumentation. The flexion, presence of a flexion contracture, or internal and external rotation at 90 degrees of flexion should all be documented in the affected extremity and presumably normal contralateral hip. In addition, fluoroscopic assessment of hip translation with gentle axial traction should be documented. Subluxation with less than 15 to 20 pounds of force is indicative of incompetent soft tissues. This patient should be considered for surgical stabilization through a combination of labral repair and/or capsular imbrication.

- Radiographic documentation of anchor position

  When performing hip labral repairs, the position of anchor placement is significantly different than in the shoulder, where most surgeons already have experience. The angle is more acute, and the soft tissues do not allow angulation of the insertion tools as easily as in the shoulder. In addition, the acetabular cavity is concave in shape, as opposed to the convexity of the shoulder. Thus, fluoroscopic confirmation of the angle of entry of the suture anchor should be obtained. Oblique images should be used in questionable cases. Any image that shows the anchor trajectory within the acetabular fossa is indicative of possible joint penetration and should prompt the surgeon to redirect it.

- Assessment of peripheral compartment

  The peripheral compartment is part of the hip joint. The area includes approximately 25% of the articular cartilage of the femur that otherwise is not seen if this compartment is not entered. More importantly, there are often LBs and sometimes labral tears, which are only seen from this vantage point. Finally, surgeons performing hip arthroscopy should be familiar with the normal variants that are seen in this compartment. When something outside the norm presents itself, the surgeon will know that there is an issue that needs to be considered in the treatment algorithm for that patient.

## PHYSICAL THERAPY

The typical capsular imbrication patient is kept partially weight bearing for 4 weeks. The critical maneuvers that must be avoided include extension and external rotation of the involved extremity. Simply making the patient non–weight bearing will cause a significant amount of stress to be borne by the hip flexor musculature and predispose the patient to problems with tendinitis. The important points with respect to the limitations in the first 4 weeks is not only extension, but most important, to limit external rotation of the affected leg. At 4 weeks, a gradual weight-bearing progression is instituted. Range of motion and strengthening of the extremity are then started, followed by full unrestricted activities beginning no earlier than 3 months postoperatively. This return is predicated on a full passive and active range of motion, as well as normal strength.

## CONCLUSION

The spectrum of hip instability is wide and includes symptomatology that ranges from what is similar to that of a simple snapping hip to a complete dislocation that results in persistent repeated dislocations or subluxations. A thorough history and physical examination, combined with the appropriate imaging studies, are essential for determining where the patient's complaints fit on this spectrum.

The treatment of these disorders also covers a wide range. Conservative care, which includes temporary immobilization, followed by activity modification, physical therapy, and the eventual return to activity, can be effective for those with mild capsular or musculotendinous injuries. More significant instability, which includes labral injury, capsular laxity, and possibly mild acetabular dysplasia, can be treated effectively with open capsular plication or, more recently, arthroscopic capsular plication and labral débridement (or repair). Hip dysplasia that involves bony abnormalities that cannot be addressed by arthroscopic or open capsular means can be treated using periacetabular osteotomy, whereas dysplasia that involves significant DJD is better treated with total hip arthroplasty. Finally, traumatic dislocations with retained LBs and/or femoral head fractures can be treated with open or arthroscopic LB removal as well as arthroscopic or open femoral head–acetabular fixation.

## REFERENCES

1. Philippon MJ. The role of arthroscopic thermal capsulorrhaphy in the hip. *Clin Sports Med.* 2001;20:817-829.
2. Takechi H, Nagashima H, Ito S. Intra-articular pressure of the hip joint outside and inside the limbus. *J Jpn Orthop Assoc.* 1982;56:529-536.
3. Ferguson SJ, Bryant JT, Ganz R, et al. An in vitro investigation of the acetabular labral seal in hip joint mechanics. *J Biomech.* 2003;36:171-178.
4. Ferguson SJ, Bryant JT, Ganz R, et al. The acetabular labrum seal: a pro-elastic finite element model. *Clin Biomech.* 2000;15:463-468.
5. Ferguson SJ, Bryant JT, Ganz R, et al. The influence of the acetabular labrum on hip joint cartilage consolidation: a pro-elastic finite element model. *J Biomech.* 2000;33:953-960.
6. Kim YT, Azuma H. The nerve endings of the acetabular labrum. *Clin Orthop.*1995;320:176-181.
7. Kelly BT, Williams RJ, Philippon MJ. Hip arthroscopy: current indications, treatment options, and management issues. *Am J Sports Med.* 2003;316:1020-1037.
8. Kallas KM, Guanche CA, Physical examination and imaging of hip injuries. *Oper Tech Sports Med.* 2002;10:176-183.
9. Scopp JM, Moorman CT III. The assessment of athletic hip injury. *Clin Sports Med.* 2001;20:647-659.
10. Hoppenfeld S. Physical examination of the hip and pelvis In: Hoppenfeld S, ed. *Physical Examation of the Spine and Extremities.* Norwalk, Conn: Appleton and Lange; 1976:143-152.
11. Tonnis D, Heinecke A, Acetabular and femoral anteversion. relationship with osteoarthritis of the hip. *J Bone Joint Surg Am.* 1999;81:747-1770.
12. Delaunay S, Dussault RG, Kaplan PA, et al. Radiographic measurements of dysplastic adult hips. *Skeletal Radiol.* 1997;26:75-81.
13. Wenger DR, Bomar JD. Human hip dysplasia: evolution of current treatment concepts. *J Orthop Sci.* 2003;8:264-271.
14. Tonnis D, Heinecke A. Acetabular and femoral anteversion: relationship with osteoarthritis of the hip. *J Bone Joint Surg Am.* 1999;81:747-1770.
15. Reynolds D, Lucas J, Klaue K. Retroversion of the acetabulum. A cause of hip pain. *J Bone Joint Surg Br.* 1999;81:281-288.
16. Edwards DJ, Lomas D, Villar RN. Diagnosis of the painful hip by magnetic resonance imaging and arthroscopy. *J Bone Joint Surg Br.* 1995;77:374-376.
17. Hodler J, Trudell D, Pathria MN, et al. Width of the articular cartilage of the hip: quantification using fat suppression spin echo MRI in cadavers. *AJR Am J Roentgenol.* 1992;192:351-355.
18. Bellabarba C, Sheinkop M, Kuo K. Idiopathic hip instability. *Clin Orthop.*1998;355: 261-271.
19. Arvidsson I. The hip joint: Forces needed for distraction and appearance of the vacuum phenomenon. *Scand J Rehabil Med.* 1990;22:157-161.
20. Crawford MJ, Dy CJ, Alexander JW, et al. The biomechanics of the hip labrum and the stability of the hip. *J Orthop Res.* 2007;465:16-22.
21. Santori N, Villar R. Acetabular labral tears: result of arthroscopic partial limbectomy. *Arthroscopy.* 2000;16:11-15.
22. Massie WK, Howorth MB. Congenital dislocation of the hip. Part 1. Methods of grading results. *J Bone Joint Surg Am.* 1950;32:519-531.
23. Tonnis D, Legal H, Graf R (eds). *Congenital Dysplasia and Dislocation of the Hip in Children and Adults.* Berlin: Springer-Verlag; 1987.
24. Lequesne M, De Seze M. [False profile of the pelvis. A new radiographic incidence for the study of the hip. Its use in dysplasias and different coxopathies.] *Rev Rheum Mal Osteoartic.* 1961;28:643-652.
25. Sanchez-Sotelo J, Berry DJ, Trousdale RT, et al. Surgical treatment of developmental dysplasia of the hip in adults: II. Arthroplasty options. *J Am Acad Orthop Surg.* 2002;210:334-344.
26. Philippon MJ, Kuppersmith DA, Wolff AB, et al. Arthroscopic findings following traumatic hip dislocation in 14 professional athletes. *Arthroscopy.* 2009;25:169-174.
27. Chudik S, Lopez V. Hip dislocations in athletes. *Sports Med Arthrosc Rev.* 2002;10:123-133.
28. Lamke LO. Traumatic dislocations of the hip. Follow-up on cases from the Stockholm area. *Acta Orthop Scand.* 1970;41:188-198.
29. Mitchell JC, Giannoudis PV, Millner PA, et al. A rare fracture-dislocation of the hip in a gymnast and review of the literature. *Br J Sports Med.* 1999;33:283-284.
30. Lieberman J, Altchek D, Salvati E. Recurrent dislocation of a hip with a labral lesion. Treatment with a modified bankart repair. *J Bone Joint Surg Am.* 1993;75:1524-1527.
31. Sullivan CR, Bickel WH, Lipscomb PR. Recurrent dislocation of the hip. *J Bone Joint Surg Am.* 1955;37:1256-1270.
32. Townsend R, Edwards G, Bazant F. Posttraumatic recurrent dislocation of the hip without fracture. *J Bone Joint Surg Br.* 51B:38-44, 1969.
33. Liebenberg F, Dommisse G. Recurrent posttraumatic dislocation of the hip. *J Bone Joint Surg Am.* 1969;51:632-637.
34. Dall D, MacNab I, Gross A. Recurrent anterior dislocation of the hip. *J Bone Joint Surg Am.* 1970;52:574-576.
35. Yamamoto Y, Takatoshi I, Ono T, Hamada Y. Usefulness of arthroscopic surgery in hip trauma cases. *Arthroscopy.* 2003;19:269-273.
36. Mullis BH, Dahners LE. Hip arthroscopy to remove loose bodies after traumatic dislocation. *J Orthop Trauma.* 20:22-26, 2006
37. Armstrong JR. traumatic dislocation of the hip: review of 101 dislocations. *J Bone Joint Surg Br.* 1948;30:430-445.
38. Brav CEA. Traumatic dislocation of the hip. *J Bone Joint Surg Am.* 1962;44:1115-1134.
39. Epstein HC. Traumatic dislocations of the hip. *Clin Orthop.* 1973;92:116-142.

## SUGGESTED READING

Martin HD, Savage A, Braly BA, et al: The function of the hip capsular ligaments: a quantitative report. *Arthroscopy.* 2008;24:188-195.

# Internal Snapping Hip Syndrome

Sunil Jani ● Marc R. Safran

A snapping hip, also referred to as coxa saltans, can be the result of external, internal, and intra-articular causes.[1-3] In 1984, Schaberg and colleagues[3] first classified the distinction between internal and external snapping hip. External snapping hip is the most common type, and is caused by the posterior iliotibial band or anterior border of the gluteus maximus slipping over the greater trochanter with hip flexion and extension. Intra-articular snapping hip can be caused by various pathologies within the hip joint, such as labral tears, loose bodies, articular cartilage flaps, displaced fracture fragments, or synovial chondromatosis.[4,5] Recently, Byrd[2] has suggested that the term *snapping hip* should only be used for extra-articular causes, because various intra-articular pathologies can be identified as causes of these symptoms.

This chapter focuses on internal snapping hip, which refers to a symptom complex most commonly attributed to catching of the iliopsoas tendon when it moves laterally to medially as the hip moves from a flexed, abducted, and externally rotated position to extension and internal rotation (Fig. 8-1).[1] In 1951, Nunziata and Blumenfeld[6] first described internal snapping tendon in a case series of three patients. Although the exact cause of the snapping remains controversial, it has been most often hypothesized to originate from the movement of the tendon over the anterior femoral head, joint capsule of the hip, or iliopectineal eminence at the pelvic brim.[2,7,8] Less commonly, the snapping may be caused by the iliopsoas tendon sliding over exostoses of the lesser trochanter.[3] Alternate theories suggest that internal snapping may be caused by the iliopsoas tendon slipping over the iliopsoas bursa—the anterior inferior iliac spine—by stenosing tenosynovitis of the iliopsoas tendon at its insertion into the lesser trochanter, or by movement of the

iliofemoral ligament over the anterior femoral head and joint capsule.[9] In actuality, it is likely that various patients may have different sources for their snapping. Different surgical approaches have been suggested for treatment based on the specific structure believed to be responsible for the snapping,[10] although it is basically a tight iliopsoas musculotendinous unit that most agree is part of the problem.

## ANATOMY

The iliopsoas muscle, composed of the psoas major and iliacus muscles, is the strongest flexor of the thigh at the hip joint. It serves as an important postural muscle and prevents hyperextension of the hip joint when standing. The iliopsoas acts inferiorly to flex the trunk when rising from a supine to a sitting position. The psoas major muscle is innervated mainly by the ventral rami of L1 and L2. It has origins on the sides of the vertebral bodies, spinous processes, and intervertebral disks from T12 to L5. The iliacus muscle is mainly innervated by the femoral nerve and originates from the superior two thirds of the iliac fossa, ala of the sacrum, and anterior sacroiliac ligaments. The iliopsoas is unique in that it has both tendinous and direct muscular attachments; it first forms from the psoas muscle superior to the inguinal ligament. As the tendon runs inferiorly, it internally rotates and fans out to insert over the lesser trochanter. The iliacus tendon joins the posterior psoas tendon at the level of the pelvic brim and inserts into the body of the femur inferior to the lesser trochanter. When the hip is flexed, the iliopsoas tendon lies lateral to the center of the femoral head–anterior hip joint capsule and iliopectineal eminence. With hip extension and

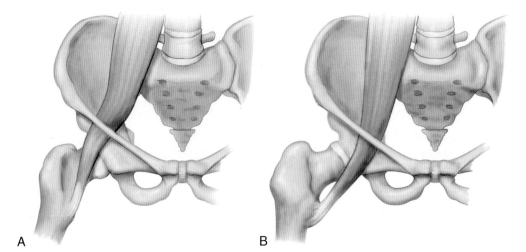

A                                                    B

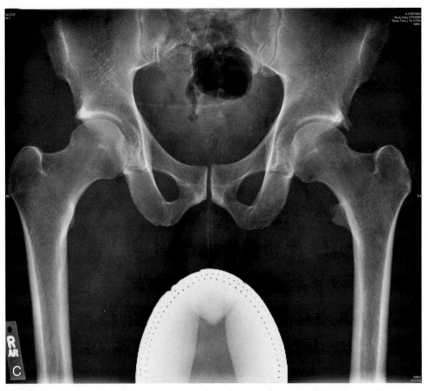

**FIGURE 8-1 A & B** *(left to right)*, The proposed mechanism of snapping iliopsoas tendon. **C,** AP pelvic radiograph of a former soccer player with a traction spur of the lesser trochanter.

internal rotation, the tendon slides across the femoral head to lie medially (see Fig. 8-1).

## HISTORY AND PHYSICAL EXAMINATION

Internal snapping hip has been estimated to exist incidentally in 5% of the population.[2] Although the snapping phenomenon is frequently asymptomatic, in certain individuals it is accompanied by pain. Certain populations, such as ballet dancers and professional athletes, are more prone to painful snapping secondary to overuse.[1,5,11,12] In one cross-sectional study, 91% of elite ballerinas reported experiencing snapping hip, with 80% having symptoms bilaterally but only 58% experiencing painful snapping. Clinical examination revealed the vast majority of these to be of the internal snapping type. The incidence of snapping hip has been noted to increase after total hip arthroplasty, often when a curved stem has been used. Usually, this can be classified as an external type of snapping hip, and it is thought to be related to catching of the posterior iliotibial band over the greater trochanter when the femoral component is placed too medially.[1] With the advent of surface replacements, and the larger femoral head component, there appears to be an increased incidence of internal snapping hip following this procedure, as compared with a standard total hip arthroplasty, because the iliopsoas snaps over a more prominent acetabular component.

With the internal and external types of snapping hip, the clinical history and physical examination are characteristically diagnostic. Snapping can often be elicited voluntarily and is reproducible. Further questioning should be directed toward determining specific activities that cause snapping in the patient.

Internal snapping hip pain can manifest as groin pain that radiates to the anteromedial thigh and/or toward the knee. A dull ache after the snapping may be reported, and can last from minutes to hours.[13] Rarely, internal snapping hip has been reported to cause pain in the lower back, flank, buttock, or sacroiliac joint.[2,14] This type of pain is related to the posterior origins of the psoas (lumbar spine) and iliacus (posterior pelvis). The patient may report a history of painless snapping that has progressed to painful snapping. Internal snapping can occur unilaterally or bilaterally, and patients may or may not report a history of trauma. For internal or external snapping hip, the reported history of trauma is often minor and/or remote, whereas an acute history of significant trauma is often associated with intra-articular pathology. With intra-articular causes for snapping, patients more often report an intermittent clicking rather than a snapping sensation.

On physical examination, internal snapping hip is characterized by a painful and often audible clunk as the patient's hip actively or passively moves from flexion, abduction, and external rotation to an extended, adducted, internally rotated position. Additional evidence to support the diagnosis of internal snapping hip can be gleaned if snapping is preceded by anterior pressure applied over the hip joint can.[1,2]

During the physical examination, it is critical to assess the patient for other causes of hip pain, including intra-articular causes. The Thomas test should be done to evaluate the patient for a flexion contracture of the iliopsoas or rectus femoris muscles. Patients may exhibit weak external rotation of the hip when it is in flexion and/or weak flexion of the hip while seated. Patients with internal snapping hip may also demonstrate an antalgic gait, most often externally rotated and abducted.[5] The patient may also have pain and/or weakness with a resisted straight leg raise with the hip flexed at 15 degrees.

## IMAGING

The diagnosis of internal snapping hip can be made exclusively from a detailed history and physical examination alone. Imaging studies may be useful in confirming the diagnosis, and are of importance in ruling out intra-articular pathology.

Plain radiographs and MRI scans are most commonly normal in patients with internal snapping hip, but they can be useful in ruling out other pathology. In patients in whom the snapping is secondary to lesser trochanter exostoses, synovial osteochondromatosis, or intra-articular loose bodies, there may be characteristic findings on plain films (see Fig. 8-1C). MRI can yield indirect evidence by demonstrating inflammation and/or swelling of the iliopsoas bursa (iliopsoas bursitis; Fig. 8-2A), or iliopsoas tendinopathy (see Fig. 8-2B). MRI is also important to rule out intra-articular causes for snapping hip, such as loose bodies and labral tears.

Iliopsoas bursography can be a used to visualize the iliopsoas tendon catching in conjunction with the patient's snapping.[3,9,15] Diagnosis of internal snapping hip can be aided by a concomitant injection of bupivacaine (Marcaine), which may provide temporarily relief of the patient's symptoms. Drawbacks to the use of iliopsoas bursography include difficulties associated with reproducing the snapping with the patient lying down constrained by the fluoroscopic imager located above the hip.[2]

The limitations of iliopsoas bursography can be overcome through the use of dynamic ultrasound to demonstrate the catching of the iliopsoas tendon.[16] This technique allows for a greater range of motion at the hip to reproduce the snapping sensation. Other evidence in support of the diagnosis of internal snapping hip includes thickening of the iliopsoas tendon and peritendinous fluid collections. A diagnostic injection of bupivacaine can also be used with dynamic ultrasound to check for alleviation of symptoms. Disadvantages of dynamic ultrasound include the fact that results are technician-dependant, and its success also requires a high-resolution ultrasound machine.[2]

## TREATMENT OPTIONS

### Conservative Management

In most cases, internal snapping hips are asymptomatic and hence require no treatment other than reassurance. Patients should be counseled that painless internal snapping is a normal variant, and is not a sign of current or future pathology. For painful internal snapping hips, the first step is activity modifi-

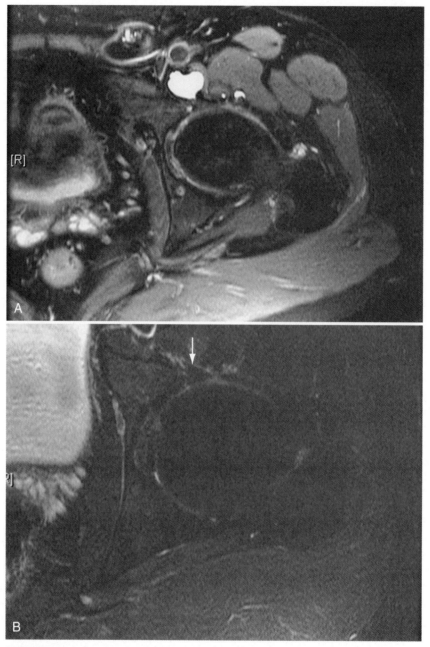

**FIGURE 8-2**  Axial cut MRI scans. **A,** Iliopsoas bursitis. Iliopsoas bursitis can accompany snapping hip. **B,** Professional tennis player with iliopsoas tendinitis. The *arrow* is pointing to the iliopsoas tendon, with the edema seen about the tendon.

cation to avoid the movements that cause pain. Additionally, physical therapy, focusing on stretching and gentle strengthening of the hip flexors and abductors, and core stabilization may prove beneficial to some patients.[1,14,17] Nonsteroidal anti-inflammatory drugs (NSAIDs) are used to decrease pain and inflammation. The vast majority of symptomatic patients are successfully treated with conservative management. However, it can take several weeks before symptoms begin to improve, and several months to 1 year before pain resolves and normal function is regained. For athletes, the goal of treatment is to be pain-free prior to returning to sports. Corticosteroid injections into the iliopsoas bursa can also be used as an adjunct for patients who do not respond to the measures described.

## Surgical Management

### Open Techniques

The persistence of painful snapping after 4 to 6 months of conservative management is an indication for surgery. The goal of surgery is to lessen the tension on the iliopsoas tendon by partially or completely releasing it. Historically, this release has been done using various open surgical techniques. These techniques have been directed at what the surgeons believed to be the main location of the snapping pathology; the methods entail releasing the tendon close it its insertion on the lesser trochanter, over the femoral head–anterior joint capsule, or near the iliopectineal eminence at the pelvic brim.[1,3,7,8,10,13] Complications associated with surgery include weakness of hip flexion, which can occur after a complete release of the tendon, and recurrence of snapping, which can occur with incomplete release, such as partial releases (lengthening of the musculotendinous unit). Furthermore, open surgical approaches endanger the lateral femoral cutaneous nerve and its branches, putting the patient at risk for loss of sensation in the anterolateral thigh.

In 1990, Jacobsen and Allen[8] published their landmark study using an open technique that involved surgical length-ening of the iliopsoas tendon via release of its posteromedial tendinous portion (Z-plasty), leaving the anterior muscle belly intact. They used a transverse inguinal incision and anterior release, based on the idea that the iliopsoas tendon is catching over the anterior femoral head and joint capsule. They performed three to four partial tenotomies beginning 1 cm proximal to the lesser trochanter, with cuts every 2 cm proximally up to the level of the femoral head, where a complete release was done at the musculotendinous junction. Twenty hips were operated on in 18 patients, and the average follow-up was 25 months. Of these hips, 70% exhibited complete resolution of snapping, and 25% had partial resolution (with decreased frequency and less pain). Overall, patients subjectively felt improvement of their symptoms in 85% of hips. Postoperative complications of this study included a 50% incidence of decreased anterolateral thigh sensation, and a 15% incidence of weakness of hip flexion. Of these cases, 10% required reoperation for persistent painful snapping.

The results for this study were included in the retrospective 20-year consecutive review published in 2004 by Hoskins and associates[18] (Table 8-1). Using the same fractional lengthening technique, data on a total of 92 hips in 80 patients were reported. The average postoperative follow-up was 6 months in their clinic and 5.4 years via telephone. Even though there was an overall complication rate of 43%, 89% of patients were satisfied with the procedure. In 22% of hips, snapping recurred after surgery, 9% of patients had decreased anterolateral thigh sensation, and 3% of patients experienced hip flexor weakness. Additional complications included one superficial infection, one hematoma, and one reoperation because of formation of a painful bursa over the lesser trochanter. Repeat tenotomies for recurring snapping resulted in heterotopic ossification in one hip and a femoral nerve palsy in another.

Taylor and Clarke[13] have reported a technique for releasing the iliopsoas tendon at the lesser trochanter using a limited (5-cm) medial incision. The iliopsoas tendon was sectioned in the interval between the pectineus and adductor brevis. The

**TABLE 8-1**    Results of Surgery for Persistent Painful Snapping of the Hip Caused by the Iliopsoas Tendon in Athletes*

| Study (Year) | No. of Hips | Elimination of Snapping (%) | Patient Satisfaction (%) | Weakness (%) | Reoperations, Decreased Sensation |
|---|---|---|---|---|---|
| Hoskins et al (2004)[18] | 92 | 78 | 89 | 3 | Reoperations (8), decreased sensation (8) |
| Gruen et al (2002)[7] | 12 | 100 | 82 | 42 | Reoperation (1) |
| Dobbs et al (2002)[10] | 9 | 89 | 100 | 0 | Decreased sensation (2) |
| Taylor and Clarke (1995)[13] | 16 | 57 | 100 | 14 | |
| *Total* | 129 | 78 | 90 | 8 | |
| Jacobsen and Allen (1990)[8] | 20 | 70 | 85 | 15 | Reoperations (2), decreased sensation (10) |
| *Total* (including Jacobson and Allen and excluding Hoskins et al) | 56 | 75 | 91 | 18 | |

*Retrospective 20-year consecutive review.
Data from Jacobson T, Allen CW. Surgical correction of the snapping iliopsoas tendon. Am J Sports Med. 1990;18:470-474.

authors hypothesized that this approach would avoid the possibility for lateral femoral cutaneous nerve injury and would provide better cosmesis. They performed their iliopsoas release 16 hips in 14 patients, with an average 17-month follow-up. All patients reported improvement in their symptoms; 57% reported complete resolution of snapping and 36% reported partial resolution of snapping. However, 14% of patients experienced postoperative weakness of hip flexion beyond 90 degrees, which was most pronounced when standing (see Table 8-1).

Dobbs and coworkers[10] have published a case series that involved fractional lengthening (Z-plasty) of the iliopsoas tendon over the iliopectineal eminence in 11 hips of nine children. The investigators performed a fractional lengthening of the tendon at the musculotendinous junction in an attempt to avoid the weakness of hip flexion that occurred in Jacobsen and Taylor and colleagues' studies.[8,13,18] They used a modified iliofemoral approach with a large 5- to 7- cm incision to allow for proper visualization and complete release of the iliopsoas tendon. The approach was meant to protect the lateral femoral cutaneous nerve, which lies medial to their plane of dissection. After an average follow-up of 4 years, all patients were satisfied with the procedure. No patients exhibited any weakness of hip flexion, and 22% of patients experienced a transient decrease of sensation in the anterolateral thigh (proposed to be caused by traction on the lateral femoral cutaneous nerve). The authors advocated immense care to distinguish the iliopsoas tendon from the nearby femoral nerve properly. In their technique, the use of paralytics was avoided and the tendon was stimulated with very low-level electrocautery prior to lengthening to confirm that no nerve fibers were associated with it. Also of note, all 9 of the children in this study had been referred with incorrect diagnoses, even though each child reliably demonstrated the palpable anterior and medial snapping over their hip that is pathognomonic for internal snapping hip (see Table 8-1).

In 2002, Gruen and associates[7] reported an open surgical technique that involved a true ilioinguinal approach and fractional lengthening (Z-plasty) of the iliopsoas tendon within the psoas muscle belly above the pelvic brim. Their study involved 12 hips in 11 patients with an average of 3 years of follow-up. All patients reported complete resolution of snapping, but 18% of patients reported that their hip pain recurred and was unchanged by surgery. Of these patients, 83% were satisfied with the pain relief that they obtained from the procedure, but 45% of patients experienced subjective weakness in hip flexion (80% of these patients only experienced weakness beyond 90 degrees of flexion). Investigators were unable to identify any weakness based on physical examination. One patient in the study underwent multiple reoperations, none of which were successful in relieving the pain (see Table 8-1).

Most complications with open iliopsoas releases may be related to one of several factors: (1) the approach used for the release can cause sensory deficits; (2) inadvertent sectioning of muscle in addition to the tendon can cause weakness of hip flexion; or (3) open releases are unable to address intra-articular pathology, which can lead to failure of the procedure and recurrence of painful snapping. As will be discussed, ar-

throscopic methods to release the iliopsoas tendon can overcome each of these issues.

## Arthroscopic Techniques

As a result of these limitations and complications of open management of internal snapping hip, arthroscopic approaches have evolved. The minimal incisions used for arthroscopic portals greatly decrease the chance for nerve injury. Arthroscopic visualization of the iliopsoas tendon allows for precise and complete release of the tendon, with very little damage to the muscle belly. Generally, the arthroscopic approach to the iliopsoas tendon comes directly on the tendon, so that direct sectioning of the tendon can be accomplished without cutting the muscle. This allows maintenance of iliopsoas function. Furthermore, the neurovascular structures at risk generally are on the opposite side of the musculotendinous unit, protected from the arthroscopic instruments by the iliopsoas muscle. Finally, during an arthroscopic iliopsoas release, diagnostic hip arthroscopy of the central and peripheral hip compartments is done to identify and address any intra-articular pathology (Fig. 8-3). Early results with arthroscopic release techniques have demonstrated that associated intra-articular injuries are present between 56% and 83% of the time.[2,19,20]

Innovations in hip arthroscopy techniques have led to the development of three different arthroscopic approaches to release the iliopsoas tendon. The procedure can be done extra-articularly within the psoas bursa at the level of the lesser trochanter, or it can be done via a trans-scapular release through either the peripheral or central compartments of the hip joint.[2,20-23]

Releasing the iliopsoas tendon from its attachment at the lesser trochanter can be done using two accessory portals in addition to the standard hip arthroscopy portals (anterolateral, posterolateral, and anterior).[2,21] On completion of hip arthroscopy on a fracture table, the instruments are removed and the traction is released. The lower extremity is placed into external rotation and the hip is flexed 15 to 20 degrees. The first accessory portal, the distal anterolateral portal, is made 2 to 3 cm distal and slightly anterior to the anterolateral portal at the level of the lesser trochanter using fluoroscopic guidance. A second accessory portal, the iliopsoas portal, is then placed 3 to 4 cm inferior to the distal anterolateral portal (Fig. 8-4A). These two portals are used for visualization of the iliopsoas tendon through the iliopsoas bursa and for instrumentation. The tendon usually appears as a bright white structure located behind the synovial tissue. To see the tendon better, a shaver can be introduced to clear adhesions and excess synovium within the bursa (see Fig. 8-4B). Once the tendon is clearly identified, it is transected directly adjacent to its insertion on the greater trochanter using an electrocautery or radiofrequency device, without incising any muscle (see Fig. 8-4C). If the tendon is transected more proximally, the medial and lateral femoral circumflex arteries may be endangered, because they wrap around the tendon 2 to 3 cm proximal to its insertion.[19] Patients should be counseled prior to surgery to expect significant weakness of their hip flexors for 2 to 4 weeks after this release. Active strengthening of hip flex-

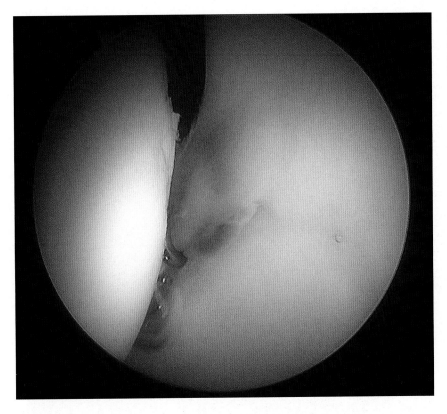

**FIGURE 8-3** Arthroscopic photograph from the anterolateral portal of the central compartment demonstrating bruising of the anterior labrum, associated with snapping hip–tight iliopsoas tendon.

ors should not begin until 6 weeks postoperatively (see Fig. 8-3).[20] Postoperatively, patients are allowed to bear weight as tolerated, using crutches, until their gait is normal. There are some anecdotal reports of heterotopic ossification with this approach, although the senior author (MRS) has not seen this in his experience. Nonetheless, consideration should be given to heterotopic bone prophylaxis post operatively.

Wettstein and colleagues[23] have described a technique to perform an iliopsoas tenotomy via a trans-scapular approach from the peripheral compartment of the hip. This technique does not require any additional portals beyond the standard hip arthroscopy portals. Following arthroscopy of the central compartment of the hip, instruments are removed, traction is released, and the hip is placed into 30 to 35 degrees of flexion, 5 to 10 degrees of abduction, and external rotation. The anterolateral and anterior portals to the peripheral compartment are then created. An arthroscope is inserted into the proximal anterolateral portal and used to identify the medial synovial fold, which is a critical landmark for this procedure. The medial synovial fold attaches distally to the lesser trochanter and bridges the anteromedial portion of the femoral head and articular joint capsule. At the level of the zona orbicularis, the medial synovial fold runs medially to the level of the iliopsoas, which is superficial to the capsule. Turning the arthroscope anteriorly, a 2-cm transverse capsulotomy is made medial to the medial synovial fold and proximal to the zona orbicularis. Here, the iliacus muscle protects the femoral neurovascular bundle and the iliopsoas tendon can be completely released (Fig. 8-5).

From the central compartment of the hip, the iliopsoas tendon is immediately medial to a thin veil of capsular tissue anterior to the joint (Fig. 8-6A). Identification of the iliopsoas tendon can be facilitated by using a probe to palpate the tendon. In cases of internal snapping hip, it is not unusual to have inflammation along the capsule adjacent to the psoas muscle and tearing or bruising of the adjacent labrum (see Fig. 8-3). Access to the tendon is made from a 1-cm capsulotomy adjacent to the anterior portal (see Fig. 8-6B). Once the tendon is identified, it is transected, leaving the overlying muscle fibers intact. When performing the iliopsoas tendon release from the central compartment, care must be taken to avoid injuring the femoral nerve that runs directly anteriorly to the iliopsoas at this level.[22]

In 2006, Byrd[2] reported preliminary results using iliopsoas tendon release at the lesser trochanter in nine patients. With an average 20-month follow-up, 100% of patients experienced complete resolution of snapping and were satisfied with the procedure. None of the patients exhibited weakness or any other complications. Of the patients, 56% were found to have concomitant intra-articular pathology that was addressed during surgery (Table 8-2).

Using the same arthroscopic technique of release of the iliopsoas tendon at the lesser trochanter, Ilizaliturri and associates[21] have demonstrated similar results in a study on seven hips in six patients. Followed for an average of 21 months, 100% of patients experienced resolution of snapping and pain and all patients were satisfied with the procedure. In this study, all patients exhibited significant weakness of hip flexion, but it was completely improved by 8 weeks. No other complications were observed. Of these patients, 57% were found to have intra-articular pathology at the time of surgery (see Table 8-2).

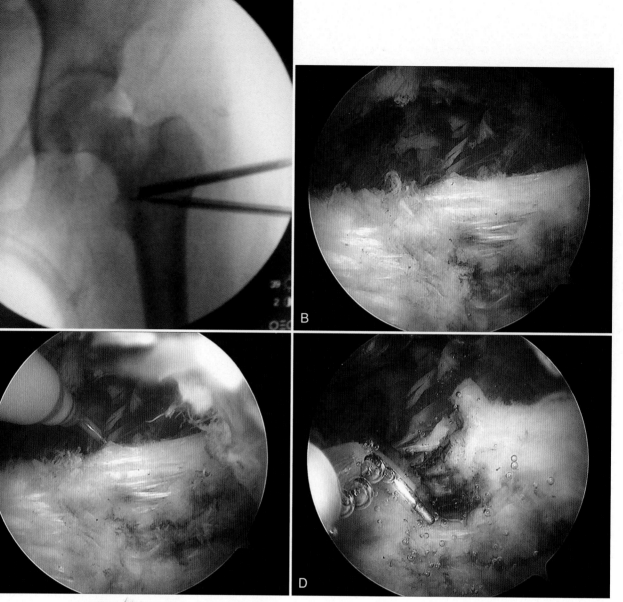

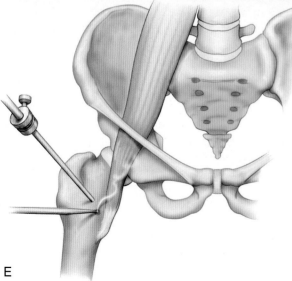

**FIGURE 8-4** Release of the iliopsoas tendon at the level of the lesser trochanter. **A,** Fluoroscopic view of the arthroscopic camera and electrocautery at the level of the lesser trochanter. **B,** Arthroscopic view of the iliopsoas tendon at the level of the lesser trochanter. **C,** Electrocautery at the tendon. **D,** Tendon being cut at the level of the lesser trochanter. **E,** Schematic representation of the iliopsoas tendon being cut arthroscopically at the lesser trochanter.

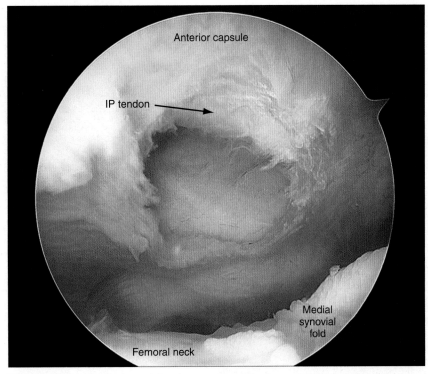

**FIGURE 8-5** Iliopsoas in the peripheral compartment; the femoral neck is below and the anterior capsule above. The medial synovial fold is seen below and to the right, and the femoral head is to the left. Out of view is the zona orbicularis, to the right. The tendon is seen through the capsulotomy.

**TABLE 8-2**    Results Using Different Arthroscopic Approaches to Iliopsoas Tendon Release

| Study (Year) | No. of Hips | Resolution of Snapping (%) | Patient Satisfaction (%) | Intra-articular Pathology (%) | Persistent Weakness (%) | Technique |
|---|---|---|---|---|---|---|
| Ilizaliturri et al (2009)[20] | 10 | 100 | 100 | 80 | NR | Lesser trochanter |
| Ilizaliturri et al (2009)[20] | 9 | 100 | 100 | 78 | NR | Transcapsular (peripheral) |
| Flanum et al (2007)[19] | 6 | 100 | 100 | 83 | 0 | Lesser trochanter |
| Byrd (2006)[2] | 9 | 100 | 100 | 56 | 0 | Lesser trochanter |
| Ilizaliturri et al (2005)[21] | 7 | 100 | 100 | 57 | 0 | Lesser trochanter |
| *Total* | 41 | 100 | 100 | 71 | 0 | |
| Wettstein et al (2006)[23] | 9 | 100 | | NR | Slight weakness observed in some (patients did not notice) | Trans-scapular (peripheral) |

*NR, Not Reported.*

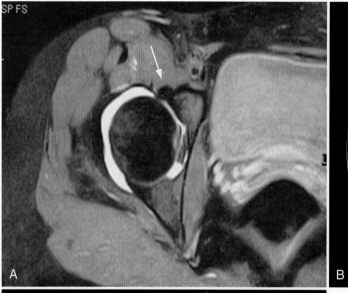

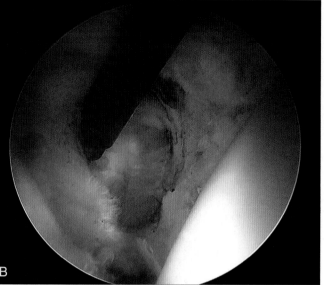

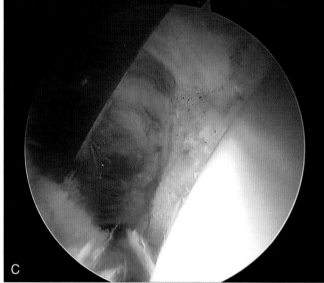

**FIGURE 8-6 A,** Axial cut MRI scan demonstrating the relationship of the iliopsoas tendon to the anterior edge of the acetabulum at the level of the joint. The tendon is adjacent to the capsule. **B,** Iliopsoas tendon after a capsulotomy is made at the anterior capsule in the central compartment. The femoral head can be seen to the right. **C,** Iliopsoas muscle after the tendon has been cut.

Flanum and coworkers[19] have published a case series of six patients with unilateral internal snapping hip confirmed by ultrasound-guided injection of the psoas bursa. All patients were treated with arthroscopic release of the iliopsoas tendon at the lesser trochanter. After 12 months of follow-up, 100% of patients had complete alleviation of painful snapping of their hips; 33% of patients reported occasional slight pain in their hips. Weakness of hip flexors was resolved in all patients by 8 weeks. Intra-articular pathology during the operation was found in 83% of patients. The mean modified Harris hip score was 58.3 preoperatively and 62.3, 84.5, 90.3, and 95.7 at 1.5, 3, 6, and 12 months respectively (see Table 8-2).

Of these 6 patients, 3 were included in a case series by Anderson and Keene[4] that investigated return to sport after arthroscopic iliopsoas tendon release in 15 athletes. Five subjects were classified as competitive athletes (2 college, 3 high school), and 10 were classified as recreational athletes. Of the 12 additional patients, 75% were found to have intra-articular pathology at the time of surgery. In this series, mean modified Harris hip scores were 41 and 44 points preoperatively for the competitive and recreational athletes, respectively. Postoperative scores were 87 and 63 at 6 weeks and 94 and 98 at 6 months. All 15 athletes had returned to participation in sports by an average of 9 months postoperatively. With an average follow-up of 17 months, all patients experienced complete alleviation of painful snapping and no recurrence. No patients experienced any weakness, decreased range of motion, sensory deficits, or other complications secondary to the surgery. There were 2 patients in these series who experienced greater trochanteric bursitis 6 weeks postoperatively because of an altered gait pattern, probably as a result of decreased power of hip flexion. This pain resolved after the patients were placed back on crutches and gradually weaned off during the subsequent 2 weeks.

In their 2006 paper detailing their technique for transscapular iliopsoas release from the peripheral hip compartment, Wettstein and colleagues reported preliminary data from nine patients. After a mean follow-up of 9 months, all patients had resolution of snapping, and no complications were reported. The incidence of intra-articular pathology was not reported. Of note, the authors mentioned that they observed "a permanent slight decrease in strength for deep hip flexion in some patients, with no subjective feeling of it."[23] Although no further data were given, this issue needs to be addressed in future studies using this technique.

Recently, Ilizaliturri and colleagues[20] published the results of a randomized clinical trial that compared the results from endoscopic release of the iliopsoas tendon at the lesser trochanter (group 1, 10 patients) and trans-scapular arthroscopic psoas release from the peripheral compartment (group 2, 9 patients). Their results demonstrated no significant clinical differences in the results between the two groups; both techniques were found to be equally effective and reproducible. Snapping and pain were 100% resolved in both groups, and there were no complications in either group. Coexisting intra-articular pathology was found in 80% of patients in group 1 and 78% of patients in group 2. Postoperative Western Ontario and McMaster (WOMAC) University osteoarthritis index scores at a minimum 1-year follow-up were not significantly different between the two groups, and both groups exhibited a statistically significant improvement from preoperative WOMAC scores. All patients in this study were given 400 mg of celecoxib daily for 21 days following surgery as prophylaxis for heterotopic ossification (HO).

To our knowledge, there have been two reports of HO occurring after surgical treatment for internal snapping hip; both of these occurred after open fractional lengthening of the iliopsoas tendon was performed through a transverse inguinal approach.[18,24] However, as noted, there has been anecdotal discussion of HO following arthroscopic iliopsoas release at the lesser trochanter.

---

**PEARLS & PITFALLS**

**PEARLS**

- Perform central compartment arthroscopy; there is up to 70% associated intra-articular pathology.
- Visualize the tendon before sectioning it.
- For peripheral compartment sectioning of the iliopsoas tendon, know arthroscopic landmarks, such as the medial synovial fold and zona orbicularis.
- For peripheral compartment cutting of the iliopsoas tendon, cut toward the arthroscope, because the artery is on the superficial surface of the overlying muscle.
- For endoscopic lengthening of the iliopsoas tendon, externally rotate and flex the femur. Using fluoroscopy, make sure that the synovium over the tendon is cleared and the tendon is well visualized.
- For endoscopic tenotomy at the lesser trochanter, keep resection at and just proximal to the lesser trochanter, because the medial and lateral circumflex vessels are 2 to 3 cm proximal to the lesser trochanter.
- For arthroscopic tenotomy at the level of the anterior acetabular rim, the level of the iliopsoas can be identified by the indentation in the anterior acetabulum
- For central compartment sectioning of the iliopsoas tendon, cut toward the arthroscope or joint, because the artery is on the superficial surface of the overlying muscle.
- Some surgeons prefer to use a knife, instead of electrocautery or radiofrequency devices, when performing the iliopsoas tenotomy at the level of the acetabulum to reduce risk to injury to the neurovascular structures.

**PITFALLS**

- Heterotopic ossification has been reported after performing an iliopsoas tenotomy at the level of the lesser trochanter.
- Cutting through the muscle overlying the iliopsoas tendon in the central and peripheral compartment may result in vascular injury.
- Not visualizing the entire circumference of the tendon may result in incomplete lengthening of the iliopsoas tendon.
- Although temporary weakness is noted after arthroscopic iliopsoas lengthening, permanent weakness has been reported with open iliopsoas lengthening and potentially could occur with the arthroscopic approach, especially with deep flexion.

## SUMMARY

Internal snapping hip is a common symptom complex that is often misdiagnosed. The keys to proper diagnosis are a high index of suspicion and a detailed history and physical examination. The snapping can be palpable along the anterior or medial hip, and it is not unusual for it to be quite loud. Imaging studies are not necessary for the diagnosis, but can aid in addressing concomitant intra-articular pathology. Internal snapping hip is often asymptomatic and does not require any formal treatment. Painful snapping is best treated non-operatively with anti-inflammatory medications and stretching of the iliopsoas, but refractory pain after 4-6 months of conservative management may benefit from surgical intervention. Arthroscopic interventions are based on similar principles to open iliopsoas releases, but early results show superior results and substantially less morbidity when performed arthroscopically. Another benefit to arthroscopic treatments is that it allows simultaneous diagnosis and treatment of any intra-articular lesions that may coexist with the snapping tendon. Arthroscopic iliopsoas releases via the peripheral hip compartment at the level of the joint capsule seem to be as effective as extra-articular release of the tendon off of the lesser trochanter. Questions remain regarding the incidence of HO in association with iliopsoas tendon releases, and whether prophylaxis is necessary.

## REFERENCES

1. Allen WC, Cope R. Coxa saltans: the snapping hip revisited. *J Am Acad Orthop Surg.* 1995;3:303-308.

2. Byrd JW. Evaluation and management of the snapping iliopsoas tendon. *Instr Course Lect.* 2006;55:347-355.

3. Schaberg JE, Harper MC, Allen WC. The snapping hip syndrome. *Am J Sports Med.* 1984;12:361-365.

4. Anderson SA, Keene JS. Results of arthroscopic iliopsoas tendon release in competitive and recreational athletes. *Am J Sports Med.* 2008;36:2263-2371.

5. Wahl CJ, Warren RF, Adler RS, et al. Internal coxa saltans (snapping hip) as a result of overtraining: a report of 3 cases in professional athletes with a review of causes and the role of ultrasound in early diagnosis and management. *Am J Sports Med.* 2004; 32:1302-1309.

6. Nunziata A, Blumenfeld I. Cadera a resorte: A proposito de una variedad. *Prensa Med Argent.* 1951;38:1997-2001.

7. Gruen GS, Scioscia TN, Lowenstein JE. The surgical treatment of the internal snapping hip. *Am J Sports Med.* 2002;30:607-613.

8. Jacobson T, Allen CW. Surgical correction of the snapping iliopsoas tendon. *Am J Sports Med.* 1990;18:470-474.

9. Harper MC, Schaberg JE, Allen WC. Primary iliopsoas bursography in the diagnosis of disorders of the hip. *Clin Orthop Relat Res.* 1987;221:238-241.

10. Dobbs MB, Gordon JE, Luhmann SJ, et al. Surgical correction of the snapping iliopsoas tendon in adolescents. *J Bone Joint Surg Am.* 2002;84:420-424.

11. Reid DC. Prevention of hip and knee injuries in ballet dancers. *Sports Med.* 1988;6:295-307.

12. Winston P, Awan R, Cassidy JD, Bleakney RK. Self-reported snapping hip syndrome in elite ballet dancers. *Am J Sports Med.* 2007; 35:118-126.

13. Taylor GR, Clarke NM. Surgical release of the "snapping iliopsoas tendon." *J Bone Joint Surg Br.* 1995;77:881-883.

14. Little TL, Mansoor J. Low back pain associated with internal snapping hip syndrome in a competitive cyclist. *Br J Sports Med.* 2008;42:308-209.

15. Vaccaro JP, Sauser DD, Beals RK. Iliopsoas bursa imaging: efficacy in depicting abnormal iliopsoas tendon motion in patients with internal snapping hip syndrome. *Radiology.* 1995;197:853-856.

16. Pelsser V, Cardinal E, Hobden R, et al. Extraarticular snapping hip: sonographic findings. *AJR Am J Roentgenol.* 2001;176: 67-73.

17. Keskula DR, Lott J, Duncan JB. Snapping iliopsoas tendon in a recreational athlete: a case report. *J Athletic Training.* 1999;34: 382-385.

18. Hoskins JS, Burd TA, Allen WC. Surgical correction of internal coxa saltans: a 20-year consecutive study. *Am J Sports Med.* 2004; 32:998-1001.

19. Flanum ME, Keene JS, Blankenbaker DG, DeSmet AA. Arthroscopic treatment of the painful "internal" snapping hip. *Am J Sports Med.* 2007;35:770-779.

20. Ilizaliturri VM Jr, Chaidez PA, Villegas P, et al. Prospective Randomized study of 2 different techniques for endoscopic iliopsoas tendon release in the treatment of internal snapping hip syndrome. *Arthroscopy.* 2009;25:159-163.

21. Ilizaliturri VM Jr, Villalobos FE Jr, Chaidez PA, et al. Internal snapping hip syndrome: Treatment by endoscopic release of the iliopsoas tendon. *Arthroscopy.* 2005;21:1375-1380.

22. Kelly BT, Williams RJ 3rd, Philippon MJ. Hip arthroscopy: current indications, treatment options, and management issues. *Am J Sports Med.* 2003;31:1020-1037.

23. Wettstein M, Jung J, Dienst M. Arthroscopic psoas tenotomy. *Arthroscopy.* 2006;22:907.

24. McCulloch PC, Bush-Joseph CA. Massive heterotopic ossification complicating iliopsoas tendon lengthening. A case report. *Am J Sports Med.* 2006;34:2022-2025.

# External Snapping Hip Syndrome

Victor M. Ilizaliturri, Jr.

The snapping hip, or coxa saltans, is characterized by a snapping phenomenon that occurs around the hip in association with hip motion. It has been classified into three different types[1]:

1. External snapping hip syndrome was the earliest type described.[2] It is caused by the iliotibial band sliding over the greater trochanter.
2. The internal snapping hip syndrome. This is caused by the iliopsoas tendon snapping over the iliopectineal eminence or the femoral head.
3. A third type, the so-called, intra-articular snapping hip, refers to intra-articular pathology causing mechanical hip symptoms (locking, catching, giving way). Because we are now more precise in the diagnosis and description of intraarticular hip pathology, the term *intra-articular snapping hip* is no longer used.[3] This chapter focuses on the external snapping hip syndrome, or coxa saltans externa.

## PATHOANATOMY

The external snapping hip syndrome is produced by a posterior thickening of the iliotibial band and an anterior thickening of fibers of the gluteus maximus. These fibers lie posterior to the greater trochanter. The thickened fibers snap on the greater trochanter with flexion and extension of the hip.

## HISTORY AND PHYSICAL EXAMINATION

The snapping phenomenon in the case of the external snapping hip syndrome is always reported by patient at the lateral upper thigh, over the area of the greater trochanter.

In some cases, the snapping phenomenon may be visible under the skin and, in some other cases, it may be palpated over the area of the greater trochanter. In symptomatic patients, the snapping phenomenon is accompanied by pain in the area of the greater trochanter. The snapping phenomenon is always voluntary and the patient often volunteers to demonstrate it.[1] Asymptomatic snapping (snapping without pain) must always be considered a normal occurrence.[4] Clinical diagnosis is evident; the snapping will occur with flexion and extension of the hip. The snapping phenomenon is also described by some patients as the ability to "dislocate the hip." This is often demonstrated by actively rotating the affected hip while tilting the pelvis in standing position. The voluntary dislocators are more frequently painless and should only be treated with stretching exercises of the iliotibial band. Symptomatic external snapping hip syndrome is always accompanied with pain and tenderness in the posterior greater trochanteric region. The pain is often secondary to greater trochanteric bursitis and may also be related to tendinosis of the trochanteric insertion of the gluteus medius. When Trendelenburg gait is also found, an associated abductor muscle tear must be suspected; this is an indication for surgical treatment.

## DIAGNOSTIC IMAGING

Anteroposterior pelvis x-rays should always be done to identify bony abnormalities, calcifications, or other pathology. The snapping phenomenon can be documented with dynamic ultrasonography and associated pathology such as tendinitis, bursitis or muscle tears can be detected.[5,6] Iliopsoas bursitis and abductor muscle tears can be diagnosed using magnetic resonance imaging (MRI).[7,8]

## TREATMENT OPTIONS

### Conservative Treatment

Most symptomatic cases improve with stretching physical therapy, nonsteroidal anti-inflammatory drugs (NSAIDs), and corticosteroid infiltration of the greater trochanter bursa.[1] When conservative treatment fails, surgical release is indicated. Open iliotibial band release or lengthening has been the traditional surgical option to treat the external snapping hip syndrome.[9-12] Recently, we have described a technique for endoscopic iliotibial band release for the treatment of external snapping hip syndrome[13] that provides access to the peritrochanteric space.

### Indications

Symptomatic external snapping hip syndrome is indicated in patients who have a snapping phenomenon over the area of the greater trochanter that occurs mainly with flexion and extension and is associated with pain and tenderness. Surgical release is indicated when conservative treatment fails.

### Contraindications

- Hip osteoarthritis requiring total hip replacement
- Local soft tissue infections
- Nonpainful snapping phenomenon over the greater trochanter
- Success of conservative treatment
- Medical contraindications for surgery

### Arthroscopic Technique

The patient is positioned laterally, similar to the setup for total hip replacement. Surgical drapes must allow for free range of motion of the lower extremity so that the snapping phenomenon is reproduced with flexion and extension of the hip. Snapping usually occurs with flexion of more than 90 degrees. Reproduction of the snapping phenomenon during surgery is important to evaluate when the release of the iliotibial band is complete (Figs. 9-1 and 9-2). No traction is necessary to access the peritrochanteric space, greater trochanteric bursa, and iliotibial band. When there is a combination of periarticular pathology and hip joint pathology, arthroscopic access to the hip joint is necessary. The patient is positioned for hip arthroscopy, preparing for traction to access the central compartment and dynamic positioning for the hip periphery. I favor the lateral position for hip arthroscopy. When arthroscopy of the hip joint is complete, the foot is taken out of the traction device, the perineal post is lowered, and the peritrochanteric space is accessed. This allows for flexion and extension for reproduction of the snapping phenomenon. A more recent positioning method for hip arthroscopy is the Spider device (Tenet Medical, Calgary, Canada) which allows for full range of motion without releasing the foot for the traction device (Figs. 9-3 and 9-4).

The greater trochanter is the main landmark for portal placement and is marked on the skin using a skin marker. I use two portals, a proximal trochanteric and distal trochanteric. The area of snapping should be between both portals to ensure that iliotibial band release will include the area that generates the problem. We also mark the area of snapping on the skin (Fig. 9-5). We start by infiltrating the space under the iliotibial band with 40 to 50 mL of saline. Next, the inferior trochanteric portal is established using a standard arthroscopic cannula that is introduced under the skin. It is directed proximally to the site of the superior trochanteric portal using the blunt obturator to develop a working space above the iliotibial band. The obturator is exchanged by a 4.0-mm 30-degree arthroscope and the inferior trochanteric portal used as the viewing portal. The site of

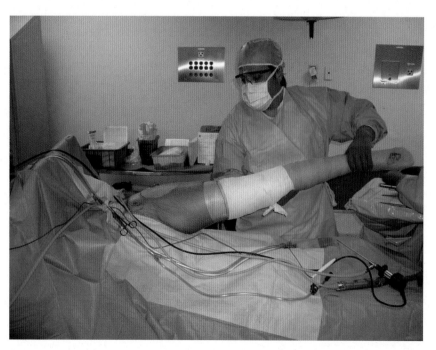

**FIGURE 9-1** Patient positioning similar to the position used for total hip replacement. This allows for full range of motion of the hip joint. In this photograph, the left hip is extended, with slight abduction and neutral rotation.

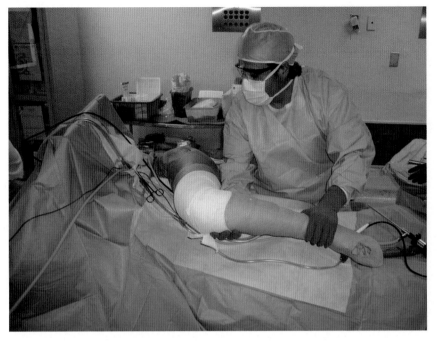

**FIGURE 9-2** Hip flexion. It is necessary to flex the hip up to 90 degrees to reproduce the snapping phenomenon.

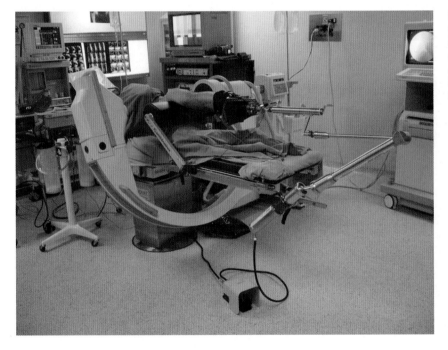

**FIGURE 9-3** Patient positioned in lateral decubitus position for arthroscopy of the left hip. Note the horizontal perineal post and the traction device attached to the Spider positioner (Tenet Medical, Alberta, Canada). The image intensifier is horizontally positioned under the table to provide an anteroposterior view of the left hip.

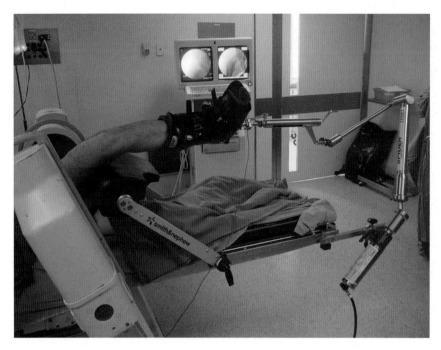

**FIGURE 9-4** By releasing the pressure of the Spider system, the hip can be flexed.

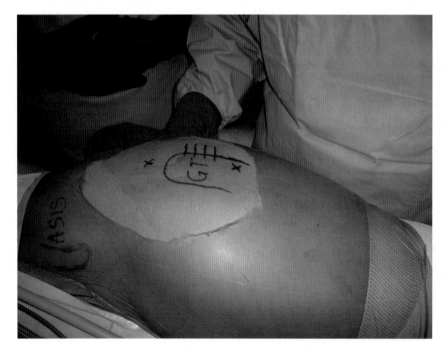

**FIGURE 9-5** Illustration of portals. The anterior superior iliac spine (ASIS) and greater trochanter (GT) have been outlined. The proximal trochanteric portal is superior to the top of greater trochanter and the distal trochanteric portal is inferior to the tip of the greater trochanter. The snapping area must be between the portals. In this case, the snapping area is indicated by horizontal lines. Note how a transparent adhesive dressing has been used to prevent fluid from accessing the patient. A portion of the transparent adhesive dressing has been removed from the surgical area to prevent plastic material to be brought in through the portals.

the proximal trochanteric portal is identified arthroscopically using a needle inserted at the portal landmark (Fig. 9-6), the skin incision is made, and a shaver is introduced to dissect subcutaneous tissue from the iliotibial band situated between the portals (Fig. 9-7). Hemostasis is performed in this step to allow clear visualization of the iliotibial band. A radiofrequency hook probe is then introduced from the proximal trochanteric portal and a 4- to 6-cm vertical retrograde cut is made on the iliotibial band starting at the level of the inferior trochanteric portal and ending at the level of the superior trochanteric portal (Fig. 9-8). The pump pressure should be kept low while working on the subcutaneous space to avoid skin complications.

Once the vertical cut on the iliotibial band is complete, the pump pressure can be increased and a transverse anterior cut of 2 cm long is made, starting at the middle of the vertical cut (Fig. 9-9). The resulting superior and inferior anterior flaps are resected using a shaver to develop a triangular defect on the anterior iliotibial band that will provide access to the posterior iliotibial band (Figs. 9-10 and 9-11). Next, a transverse posterior cut is started at the same level of the transverse anterior cut. This is the most important release and should be carried out until the snapping phenomenon is eliminated. Finally, the superior and inferior posterior flaps are resected, which results in a diamond-

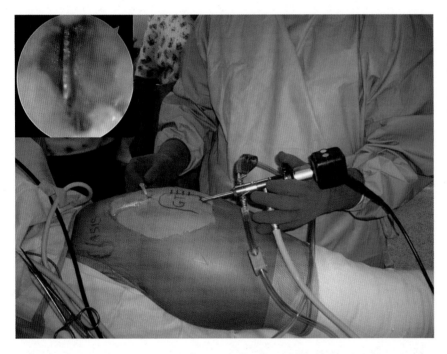

**FIGURE 9-6** A 4-mm 30-degree arthroscope is positioned above the iliotibial band at the subcutaneous space from the distal trochanteric portal. A needle is at the site of the proximal trochanteric portal. **Insert,** Arthroscopic photograph demonstrating endoscopic visualization of the needle at the proximal trochanteric portal.

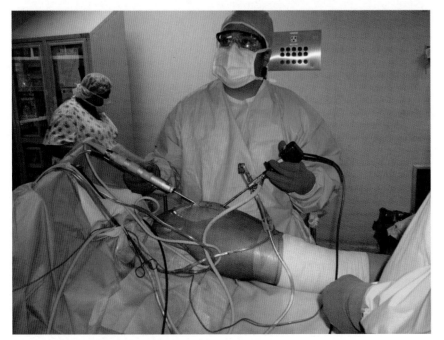

**FIGURE 9-7** The arthroscope is at the distal trochanteric portal and a mechanical shaver is at the proximal trochanteric portal.

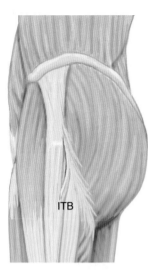

**FIGURE 9-8** Vertical cut of the iliotibial band (ITB) above the area of the greater trochanter on a left hip.

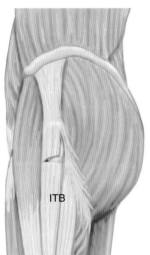

**FIGURE 9-9** Anterior transverse cut at the midportion of the anterior margin of the vertical cut on the iliotibial band (ITB) on a left hip.

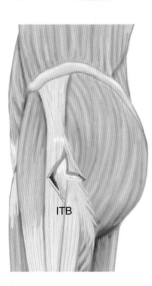

**FIGURE 9-10** Anterior triangular defect of the iliotibial band (ITB) after the superior and inferior flaps of the anterior transverse cut are resected on a left hip.

<hr>

**PEARLS&PITFALLS**

**PEARLS**

- Hypotensive anesthesia control is critical for visualization in the subcutaneous and peritrochanteric space. Inform the anesthesiologist preoperatively that the systolic pressure should remain below 100 mm Hg.
- When doing an iliotibial band release for external snapping hip syndrome, it is very important to identify the snapping phenomenon with the patient anesthetized and in the surgical position. The snapping should be between the endoscopy portals for an adequate release.
- The snapping may be very apparent and visually identified though the skin, or identified only by palpation of the greater trochanteric region.
- The posterior aspect of the iliotibial band can be visualized endoscopically snapping over the posterior part of the greater trochanter once the anterior releases have been completed.
- The first step of this technique is performed in the subcutaneous space. To prevent complications, the pump pressure must be kept low (20 to 30 mm Hg). Use inflow only when carrying out the procedure; close inflow when changing instruments. Once the first vertical cut on the iliotibial band is completed, the pump pressure may be elevated to 50 mm Hg because the fluid will be accommodated in the thigh compartment or lost through leakage from the portals. It is important to close the inflow when changing instruments or evaluating snapping to make fluid management more efficient.
- Abduction of the hip may prevent injury to the abductor tendons while performing the first release. Infiltration of 60 mL of saline under the iliotibial band, before the procedure starts, may help increase the space between the iliotibial band and greater trochanter further.
- Visualization of the iliotibial band and the peritrochanteric space must be optimal. I prefer to use an ablation design radiofrequency device for hemostasis throughout the procedure. Careful hemostasis will also prevent the formation of postoperative hematomas.
- The radiofrequency hook probe, shaver, and ablation device are interchanged throughout the procedure; a slotted cannula may be used to facilitate the exchange.
- Aspirate the fluid from the peritrochanteric space when the procedure is finished.

**PITFALLS**

- The posterior transverse release of the iliotibial band treats the snapping phenomenon of the external snapping hip syndrome. Insufficient posterior release will result in recurrence. The most posterior part of the release should be performed under clear visualization from under the iliotibial band and in retrograde fashion using a radiofrequency hook probe. This technique will prevent damage to the sciatic nerve and structures within the paratrochanteric space.
- Resection of the greater trochanteric bursa should be performed carefully to protect the underlying gluteus medius tendon. Using the shaver with the cutting window oriented on its side, over the greater trochanteric bursa facing the camera, will protect the medius tendon.

shaped defect on the iliotibial band (Figs. 9-12 and 9-13). The greater trochanter will rotate freely within the defect without snapping. The greater trochanteric bursa should be removed through the defect on the iliotibial band and the abductor tendons inspected for tears (Fig. 9-14).

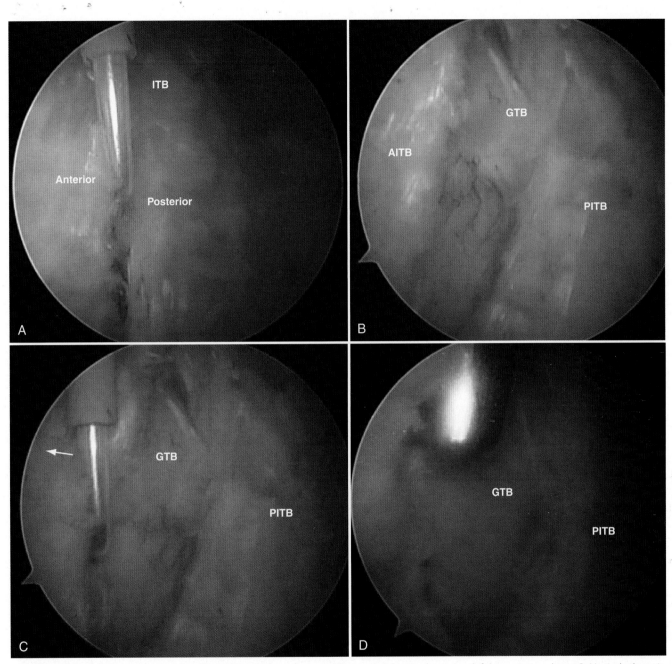

**FIGURE 9-11** Endoscopic sequence of an iliotibial band release for external snapping hip syndrome in a left hip, anterior release. **A,** Vertical release is performed, resulting in anterior and posterior margins of the iliotibial band (ITB). **B,** When the vertical release is complete the greater trochanteric bursa (GTB) is visible through the defect between the anterior margin of the iliotibial band (AITB) and the posterior margin of the iliotibial band (PITB). **C,** Direction of the anterior cut at the midportion of the vertical release on the anterior margin of the iliotibial band (*arrow*). The GTB and PITB are observed behind the radiofrequency hook. **D,** A mechanical shaver is used to resect the superior and inferior flaps after the anterior transverse release is completed. Note the triangular defect on the iliotibial band. The GTB is visible through the defect. To the right is the PITB.

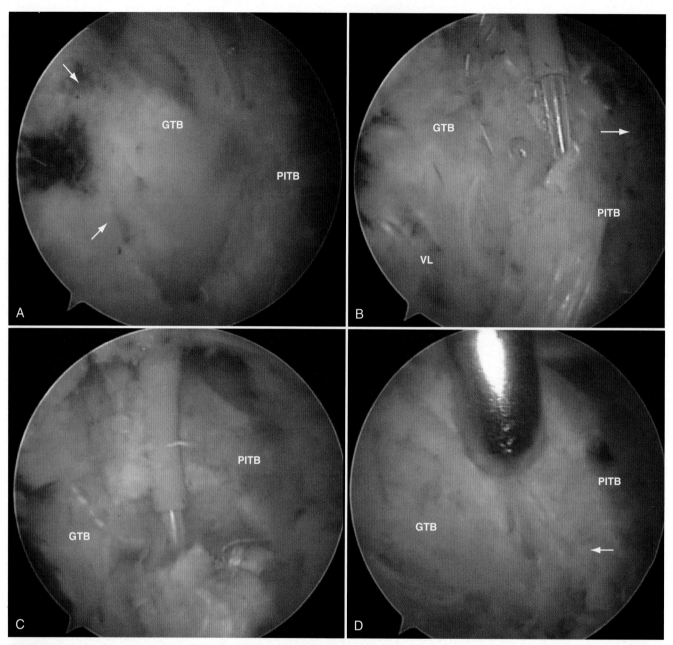

**FIGURE 9-12** Endoscopic sequence of an iliotibial band release for external snapping hip syndrome in a left hip, posterior release. **A,** Triangular defect is observed on the iliotibial band after the flaps forming the anterior transverse cut have been removed. The edges of the anterior release can be seen (*arrows*). The greater trochanteric bursa is visible through the defect and the posterior margin of the iliotibial band (PITB) is the base of the triangular defect. **B,** Radiofrequency hook probe used to perform the posterior transverse release at the midportion of the PITB. The direction of the cut is shown (*arrow*). The greater trochanteric bursa (GTB) and some fibers of the vastus lateralis (VL) are observed through the defect. **C,** The posterior transverse release of the PITB is complete. The greater trochanteric bursa is visible through the defect. **D,** Shaver is used to remove the superior and inferior flaps of the posterior transverse release on the PITB. The apex of the posterior release forming the posterior tip of the diamond-shaped defect can be seen (*arrow*). The GTB is observed through the defect.

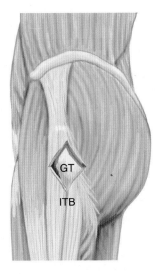

**FIGURE 9-13** Diamond-shaped defect on the iliotibial band (ITB) after release for external snapping hip syndrome. The greater trochanter (GT) is observed through the defect on a left hip.

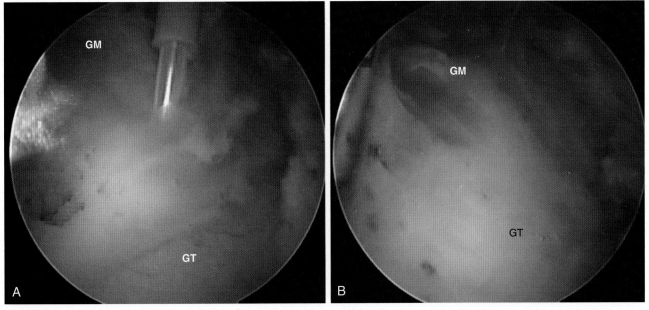

**FIGURE 9-14** Endoscopic photographs demonstrating a greater trochanteric bursectomy of a left hip. **A,** The greater trochanteric bursa is removed using a radiofrequency hook probe. The area is visualized and accessed though a diamond-shape released of the iliotibial band. The greater trochanter (GT) covered by the insertion of gluteus medius and vastus lateralis is at the bottom. Distal fibers of the gluteus medius (GM) are observed through the bursa at the top. **B,** After resection of the greater trochanteric bursa, the insertion of the GM is clearly observed on the GT. No tears are seen.

**TABLE 9-1**  Results of Surgical Treatment of External Snapping Hip Syndrome

| Study (Year) | No. of Hips | Technique | Follow-up | Pain | Resnapping |
|---|---|---|---|---|---|
| Fery and Sommelet (1988)[12] | 35 | Open, cross-cut, and inverted flap suture | 7 yr | 21 cases | 10 cases |
| Faraj et al (2001)[10] | 11 | Open, Z-plasty | 12 mo | 3 cases | 0 |
| Provencher et al (2004)[4] | 9 | Open, Z-plasty | 22 mo | 1 | 0 |
| White et al (2004)[9] | 17 | Open vertical incision and multiple transverse cuts | 32.5 mo | 0 | 2 cases (reoperated) |
| Ilizaliturri et al (2006)[13] | 11 | Diamond-shaped defect | 25 mo | 0 | 1 case, improved with physical therapy |

## RESULTS

Published literature on the results of surgical treatment of the external snapping hip syndrome is limited. Most reports have been about open releases of the iliotibial band and the evidence is anecdotal.[9-12] Recently, our group reported the results of an endoscopic technique to release the iliotibial band with greater trochanteric bursectomy and examination of the abductor tendons.

A summary of the results of open and endoscopic techniques for iliotibial band release in the treatment of external snapping hip syndrome is presented in Table 9-1. There is little information about the results of the endoscopic technique, but they compare well with the reported results of open surgical procedures.

## REHABILITATION

Range of motion of the hip or knee joints is not restricted after an endoscopic release of the iliotibial band for the treatment of external snapping hip syndrome. The patient is instructed to walk with crutches or a walker for 3 weeks after the procedure, with the ipsilateral foot flat on the floor and with partial weight bearing to avoid postoperative pain secondary to the iliotibial band release. When a rupture of the gluteus medius or minimus is associated with the snapping phenomenon, crutches or walkers are also recommended, with foot-flat and partial weight bearing to protect the abductor repair.

In the absence of abductor muscle lesions, active range of motion and strength exercises are usually started 3 weeks after the procedure. Patients return to activities of daily living by the fourth week postoperative and participation in athletic activity is usually possible by 6 to 8 weeks. In the case of associated abductor tears, activities of daily living are usually possible at 6 to 8 weeks and the return to athletic activity depends on each patient.

## CONCLUSIONS

Only recently has endoscopic management of symptomatic external snapping hip syndrome been reported.[13] I have found this procedure to be safe and reproducible. Appropriate patient selection is an important factor for ensuring good results of surgical treatment.

## REFERENCES

1. Allen WC, Cope R. Coxa saltans: the snapping hip revisited. *J Am Acad Orthop Surg.* 1995;3:303-308.
2. Binnie JF. Snapping hip (Hanche a resort; Schnellend Hefte). *Ann Surg.* 1913;58:59-66.
3. Byrd JWT. Evaluation and management of the snapping iliopsoas tendon. *Tech Orthop.* 2005;20:45-51.
4. Provencher MT, Hofmeister EP, Muldoon MP. The surgical treatment of external coxa saltans (the snapping hip) by Z-plasty of the iliotibial band. *Am J Sports Med.* 2004;32:470-476.
5. Pelsser V, Cardinal E, Hobden R, et al. Extra-articular snapping hip:sonographic findings. *AJR Am J Roentgenol.* 2001;176:67-73.
6. Choi YS, Lee SM, Song BY, Paik SH, Yoon YK. Dynamic sonography of external snapping hip syndrome. *J Ultrasound Med.* 2002;21:753-8.
7. Wunderbaldinger P, Bremer C, Schellenberger E, et al. Imaging features of iliopsoas bursitis. *Eur Radiol.* 2002;12:409-415.
8. Cvitanic O, Henzie G, Skezas N, et al. MRI diagnosis of tears of the hip abductor tendons (gluteus medius and gluteus minimus). *AJR Am J Roentgenol.* 2004;182:137-43.
9. White RA, Hughes MS, Burd T. A new operative approach in the correction of external coxa saltans. *Am J Sports Med.* 2004; 32:1504-1508.
10. Faraj AA, Moulton A, Sirivastava VM. Snapping iliotibial band. Report of ten cases and review of the literature. *Acta Orthop Belg.* 2001;67:19-23.
11. Brignall CG, Stainsby GD. The snapping hip. Treatment by Z-plasty. *J Bone Joint Surg Br.* 1991;73:253-254.
12. Fery A, Sommelet J. The snapping hip. Late results of 24 surgical cases. *Int Orthop.* 1988;12:277-82.
13. Ilizaliturri VM Jr, Martinez-Escalante FA, Chaidez PA, Camacho-Galindo J. Endoscopic iliotibial band release for external snapping hip syndrome. *Arthroscopy.* 2006;22:505-510.

# Abductor Tears

Asheesh Bedi ● Bryan T. Kelly

Disorders of the peritrochanteric compartment of the hip, including trochanteric bursitis, external coxa saltans, and abductor tears, are not uncommon and have collectively been categorized as greater trochanteric pain syndrome (GTPS). Although the mainstay of treatment of these disorders is primarily nonsurgical, patients with intractable symptoms have conventionally required open surgery. As surgeons have become increasingly adept with minimally invasive techniques, arthroscopic treatment of peritrochanteric compartment disorders of the hip has increasingly been described.

Tendinopathy and tears of the gluteus medius and minimus tendons are a common cause of recalcitrant pain along the lateral side of the hip. Tears of the gluteus medius and minimus tendon were first described by Bunker and Kagan and colleagues in the late 1990s.[1,2] Bunker and associates[1] reported a 22% incidence of concomitant medius tears in 50 patients treated for femoral neck fractures. The tears were most commonly seen distally at the junction of the gluteus medius and minimus. Howell and coworkers[3] reported that 22% of women and 16% of men who underwent total hip arthroplasty for osteoarthritis (N = 176) had abductor tears. The incidence was greater with increased age in both groups.

Abductor tears should certainly be suspected in patients with intractable GTPS in whom conservative management has failed. The pain can be variable, but is characteristically exacerbated by weight-bearing and resisted hip abduction. Bird and colleagues[4] used MRI to evaluate the integrity of the gluteus medius in 24 women with recalcitrant GTPS. A tear of the medius tendon insertion was found in 46% of patients, and an additional 38% had gluteus medius tendonitis without an appreciable tear. Kagan and associates[2] performed an open medius tendon repair in 7 patients with recalcitrant GTPS and magnetic resonance imaging (MRI) evidence of a tear. In all cases, the tear was located anteriorly in the lateral facet portion of the insertion. Repairs were performed using bone tunnels and anchors. At a median follow-up of 45 months, all patients were pain-free and all but one returned to previous levels of activity.

Although the causes of these tears are likely multifactorial, gluteus medius and minimus tears likely reflect a progressive degenerative process. A precipitating traumatic event is possible but uncommon. Most patients describe an insidious but often debilitating lateral-sided hip pain. The abductors have been likened to the rotator cuff of the hip, with the medius and minimus tendon analogous to the supraspinatus and subscapularis muscles. The medius tendon inserts on the lateral and posterosuperior facets, resulting in a moment arm similar in direction and force to the supraspinatus. The minimus inserts on the anterior facet and, depending on the position of the femur, can exert several different moments, including flexion, abduction, and internal and external rotation. Based on these observations, it follows that one of the primary functions of the minimus is to act as a head stabilizer. However, in many functional flexion angles, it provides a primary internal rotation force similar to that of the subscapularis.[5] Similar to the rotator cuff, tears of the medius are significantly more common than those of the minimus. It has been estimated that almost 25% of middle-aged women and 10% of middle-aged men will develop a tear of the gluteus medius tendon.[3,6] Tears are four times more common in women than in men.

Medius tears can be characterized as full-thickness, partial-thickness, or interstitial. These tears likely reflect a continuous spectrum of pathology, with progression from partial-thickness to full-thickness tears occurring over time.

Tear progression appears to occur by degeneration of the undersurface propagating posteriorly into a full-thickness tear.[3,6] Most tears occur in the anterior portion of the tendon as it attaches into the lateral facet of the greater trochanter. These frequently start as partial-thickness undersurface tears that propagate into full-thickness lesions that can extend posteriorly.

Both open and arthroscopic techniques of repair can provide excellent symptomatic relief and restore abductor function. Arthroscopic techniques provide a less invasive alternative and can be readily performed. Regardless of the technique, however, determining the anatomic gluteus medius footprint is critical and can often be difficult. Unlike the supraspinatus tendon, no articular margin is present to be used as a reference landmark.[6]

## ANATOMY

The peritrochanteric space is a well-defined compartment between the greater trochanter and iliotibial band and is occupied by the trochanteric bursa. Its borders are defined by (1) proximal sartorius and tensor fascia lata muscles anteriorly, (2) vastus lateralis inferomedially, (3) anterior tendon of the gluteus maximus inserting into the iliotibial band distally, and (4) gluteus medius and minimus tendons superomedially.

The gluteus medius tendon has two separate entheses on the greater trochanter. The posterior fibers attach to the posterosuperior facet (PSF), whereas the central and anterior fibers insert on the lateral facet (LF) of the trochanter. The facets are oriented at different planes relative to one another (Figs. 10-1 and 10-2).[7] The tendinous portion inserting into the PSF is robust, with a circular insertion site of approximate radius of 8.5 mm. The surface area of this insertion is approximately 200 mm$^2$. The lateral facet insertion is more rectangular in shape, with a surface area approximating 440 mm$^2$.

The trochanteric insertion of the gluteus minimus is separated from the proximal portion of the LF footprint by the trochanteric bald spot. Near the midsubstance of the LF footprint, the bald spot ends and the long head of the minimus begins. At this location, the medius footprint abuts and covers a portion of the gluteus minimus.[7] The trochanteric bald spot is circular in shape, with a radius of approximately 11 mm. Although it combines with the gluteus medius to comprise the entire lateral facet of the greater trochanter (see Fig. 10-1 and 2), it is critical not to overestimate the size of tendon detachment with an abductor tear by mistakenly incorporating the normal bald spot into the anatomic footprint of the medius tendon.[6]

The anatomically distinct insertions of the medius are thought to correlate with anatomically distinct portions that function in a phasic manner during the gait cycle. The posterior portion that inserts into the PSF is thought to stabilize the femoral head in the acetabulum during heel strike. The central portion, inserting into the PSF and LF junction, runs more vertically and is thought to be critical in initiating hip abduction. The anterior portion aids in abduction but also functions as an external rotator of the pelvis during swing-through on the contralateral limb.[7]

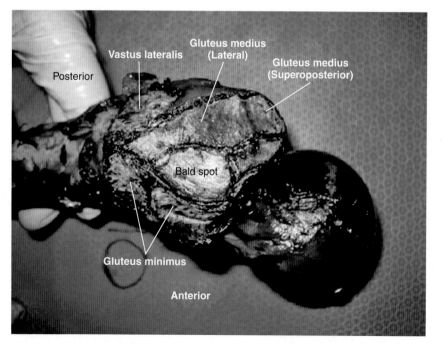

**FIGURE 10-1** Cadaveric dissection of greater trocanther demonstrating gluteus medius insertion footprints at the superoposterior (SP) and lateral facets, and their relationship to the vastus tubercle and gluteus minimus insertion. There is a bald spot that lies between the insertion of the gluteus medius on the lateral facet and the insertion of the gluteus minimus on the anterior facet. *(From Robertson WJ, Gardner MJ, Barker JU, et al. Anatomy and dimensions of the gluteus medius tendon insertion. Arthroscopy. 2008;24:130-136.)*

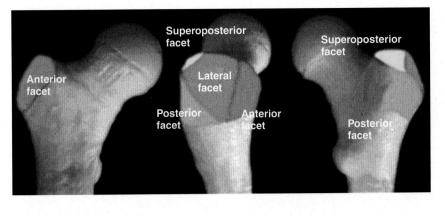

**FIGURE 10-2** The greater trochanter has been divided into four anatomical facets by Dwek and colleagues—superoposterior, lateral, anterior, and posterior. The medius inserts on the superoposterior and lateral facets, whereas the minimus attaches to the anterior facet. The posterior facet is covered by the trochanteric bursa. *(From Dwek J, Pfirrman C, Stanley A, et al. MR imaging of the hip abductors: normal anatomy and commonly encountered pathology at the greater trochanter.* Magn Reson Imaging Clin North Am. *2005;13:691-704.)*

## CLASSIFICATION

Dwek and associates[8] and others[9-14] have described a standardized MRI approach to abductor tear classification. They have divided the greater trochanter into four facets—posterosuperior, lateral, anterior, and posterior (Fig. 10-3; see Fig. 10-2). The minimus attaches to the anterior facet (see Fig. 10-3A and B). Figure 10-3A shows the normal attachment of the minimus and Figure 10-3B shows the corresponding image demonstrating a gluteus minimus tear. The medius inserts on the lateral and posterosuperior facets (see Figs. 10-3C-F). Figures 10-3C and E show the normal insertional anatomy of the medius on the LF and PSF whereas Figures 10-3D and F show corresponding images demonstrating medius tendon tears at the respective facets. The posterior facet is covered by the trochanteric bursa (see Fig. 10-3G) .

## SURGICAL TECHNIQUE

Entry into the peritrochanteric space or lateral compartment typically follows routine evaluation and treatment of pathology in the central and peripheral compartments. Central compartment arthroscopy is used for all patients who have peritrochanteric space endoscopy to document and treat any associated intra-articular pathology that may coexist with the lateral-sided pathology.

As with any arthroscopic procedure, portal placement is critical. The technique begins with accurate identification of the trochanter and anterior superior iliac spine. The anterior or midanterior portals can afford access into the peritrochanteric space. The anterior portal is placed 1 cm lateral to the anterosuperior iliac spine (ASIS) in the interval between the tensor fascia lata (TFL) and sartorius (Fig. 10-4). We prefer, however, to use a midanterior portal rather than a direct anterior portal. This is typically located 2 to 3 cm distal and 2 to 3 cm lateral to a standard anterior portal, and can be located by creating an equilateral triangle between the anterior and lateral portals.[6] It lies directly anterior to the lateral prominence of the greater trochanter and provides the safest access to the joint by avoiding any potential injury to the more proximal gluteus medius musculature and the more distal vastus lateralis musculature. It also offers an improved angle of approach to the peritrochanteric space and minimizes risk of injury to the lateral femoral cutaneous nerve compared with a direct anterior portal. Care should be taken to avoid placing the midanterior portal too proximally or distally. A proximally misplaced portal will injure the gluteus medius belly, whereas a distally misplaced portal will injure the vastus lateralis. The use of fluoroscopic imaging can confirm placement of the portal directly over the lateral prominence of the greater trochanter and prevent inadvertent proximal or distal muscular injury.

The cannula is directed into the peritrochanteric space in an anterior to posterior direction, with the leg in full extension, held in 0 degrees of adduction, 10 degrees of flexion, and 15 degrees of internal rotation (see Fig. 10-4).[6] Traction is released prior to entry into the lateral space to relax tension on the iliotibial band. Slight abduction may also be necessary to increase the space between the iliotibial band and greater trochanter. A gentle axial load may be applied if it is difficult to distinguish the muscular fibers of the gluteus medius from the overlying bursal tissue. The cannula is swept back and forth between the iliotibial band and trochanteric bursa, using a technique similar to that used for access into the subacromial space of the shoulder. The iliotibial band is analogous to the coracoacromial ligament of the shoulder.

When the appropriate plane is identified, a clear space between the iliotibial band and greater trochanter can be easily identified (Fig. 10-5A). Typically, bursal tissue is present in the space and can be easily cleared with a motorized shaver to define the lateral (iliotibial band) and medial (greater trochanter and vastus lateralis) borders of the space more clearly (see Fig. 10-5B). With the camera focus directed distally, a distal anterolateral accessory (DALA) portal in the peritrochanteric space is established with spinal needle guidance approximately 4 to 5 cm distally and in line with the anterolateral portal. This portal allows for further distal access for diagnostic and operative intervention and provides outflow (see Fig. 10-4).[6] A standard anterolateral portal can also be useful as a third working or viewing portal placed just proximally to the anterolateral tip of the greater trochanter. This portal can improve distal visualization and facilitate suture management with abductor repair.

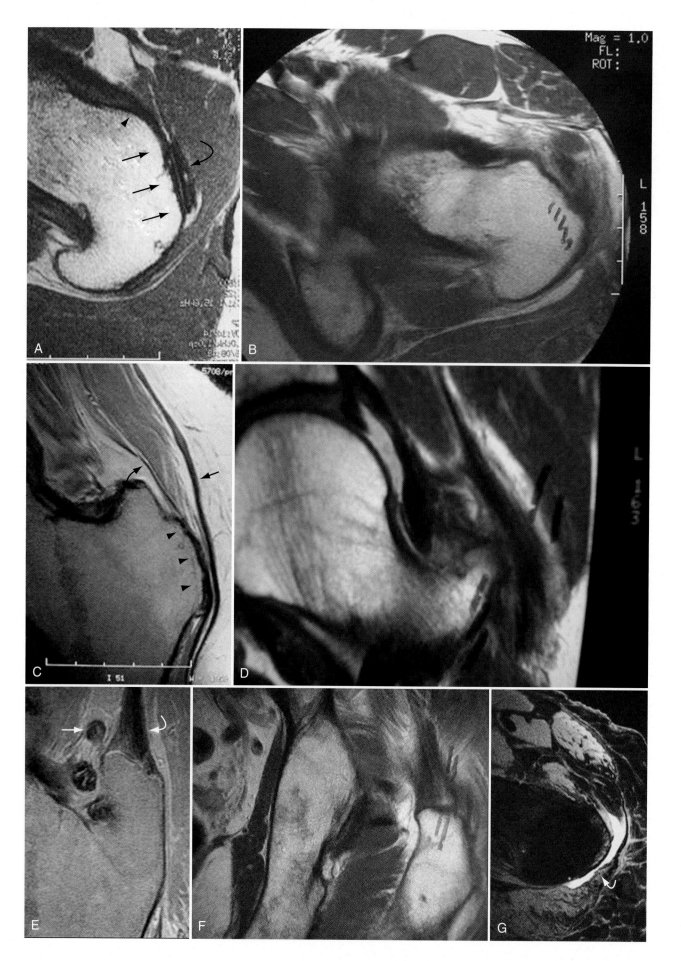

**FIGURE 10-3 A,** Axial MRI scan demonstrating the anterior facet (*straight arrows*) and inserting minimus tendon (*curved arrow*). **B,** Similar axial view demonstrating abnormal signal characteristics in the inserting tendon consistent with a high-grade partial tear. **C,** Coronal MRI scan demonstrating the lateral facet (*arrowheads*) and inserting medius tendon (*arrow*). **D,** The anterior fibers of the gluteus medius insertion onto the lateral facet are partially torn in this coronal image. **E,** Coronal MRI scan demonstrating the posterosuperior facet and the more robust tubular insertion of the medius tendon (*curved white arrow*). **F,** In this coronal image, there is evidence of partial tearing of the most lateral fibers of the posterosuperior medius insertion. **G,** Axial MRI scan demonstrating the posterior facet (*curved white arrow*). This is the only facet without a distinct tendon insertion and is the location of the trochanteric bursae. *(From Dwek J, Pfirrman C, Stanley A, et al. MR imaging of the hip abductors: normal anatomy and commonly encountered pathology at the greater trochanter. Magn Reson Imaging Clin North Am. 2005;13:691-704.)*

Diagnostic arthroscopy is initiated with the 70-degree arthroscope in the midanterior portal. The first structure visualized is the gluteus maximus inserting on the femur just below the vastus lateralis. This is a reproducible landmark and no exploration should be performed posterior to the tendon, because the sciatic nerve lies within close proximity (2 to 4 cm) to this location. Inspection then proceeds in a counterclockwise direction, starting distally and poste-

rior at the gluteus maximus insertion and then proceeding proximally and anterior toward the vastus lateralis and gluteus minimus (Fig. 10-6).[6]

As the arthroscope is moved proximally, the longitudinal fibers of the vastus lateralis are identified and traced up to the vastus tubercle, looking immediately anterior to the lateral facet (Fig. 10-7).[6] The gluteus medius tendon and muscle are best visualized at the lateral facet with the arthroscope in the proximal anterolateral portal, with the light source rotated to visualize anteriorly and superiorly (Fig. 10-8A). Visualization of the gluteus minimus can be difficult because it is usually covered by muscle tissue of the gluteus medius. By gently sweeping away medius muscle, the tendinous insertion of the minimus onto the anterior facet can be visualized (see Fig. 10-8B). Fibrous bands in this area will require excision. Hemostasis can be obtained with radiofrequency ablation or standard cautery. The fibers of the medius lie posterior to the minimus and should be carefully probed to inspect for a tear (see Fig. 10-8C). Finally, the arthroscope should be directed toward the iliotibial band. The posterior third of the iliotibial band may demonstrate abrasive changes if a symptomatic coxa saltans externus is present. An arthroscopic release can be performed if necessary (Fig. 10-9).[15] The working instruments can be placed in the midanterior and distal anterolateral accessory portals if an abductor repair or iliotibial band release is necessary.

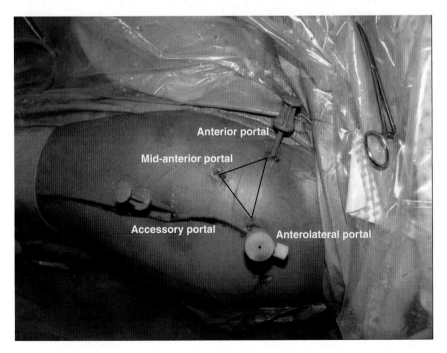

**FIGURE 10-4** Portals used for peritrochanteric arthroscopy and medius tear arthroscopic repair. Note the equilateral triangular relationship between the direct anterior, midanterior, and anterolateral portals. The distal (accessory) portal (distal anterolateral accessory) is in line with the anterolateral portal and is placed midway between the tip of the greater trochanter and the vastus tubercle, approximately 3 to 4 cm distally. *(From Voos JE, Rudzki JR, Shindle MK, et al. Arthroscopic anatomy and surgical techniques for peritrochanteric space disorders in the hip. Arthroscopy. 2007;23:1246.)*

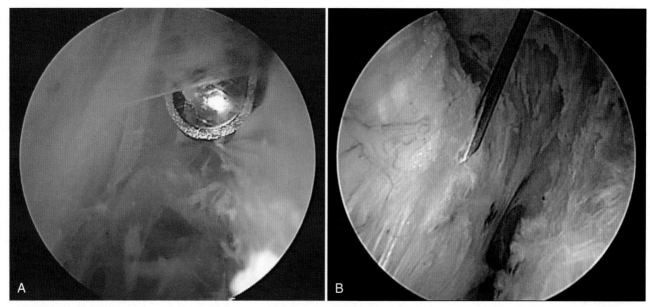

**FIGURE 10-5 A,** A blunt trochar is swept back and forth to develop the space between the iliotibial band and trochanteric bursa, using a technique similar to that for access to the subacromial space of the shoulder. **B,** Once the space is developed and cleared of bursal tissue, the greater trochanter (being touched by the spinal needle) and iliotibial bands (*right*) can be clearly identified. The greater trochanter is analogous to the greater tuberosity in the shoulder and the iliotibial band is analogous to the coracoacromial ligament.

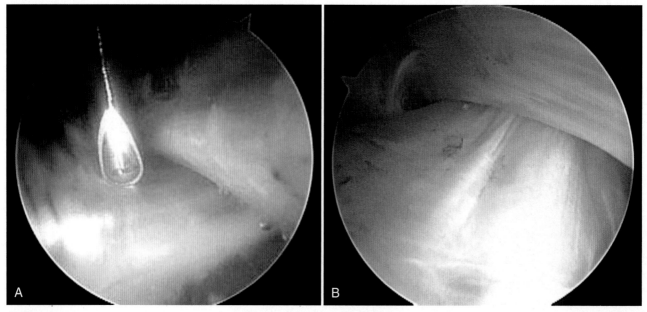

**FIGURE 10-6** The initial view identifies the so-called sickle band, or insertion of the gluteus maximus running posterior to the vastus lateralis toward the iliotibial band and posterior femur. **A,** Viewed from the anterolateral portal looking distal, the maximus tendon insertion can be cleared of tissue and serves as a distal landmark. It is typically unnecessary to extend any surgical dissection distal to this tendon insertion. **B,** When viewed from the distal anterolateral accessory portal, the tendon insertion can be closely inspected. The sciatic nerve lies approximately 3 to 4 cm posterior to the maximus insertion. Instruments should not be placed posterior to the maximus insertion without direct visualization to make sure that the nerve is protected.

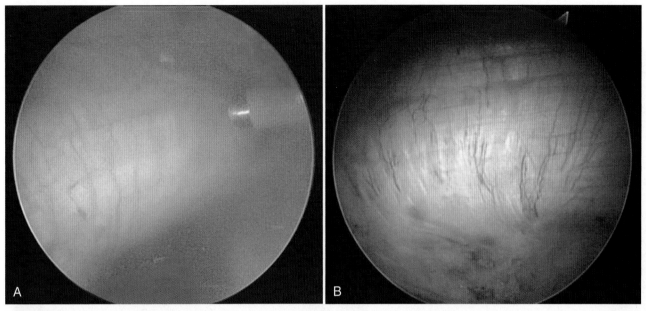

**FIGURE 10-7** As the arthroscope is moved proximally, the longitudinal fibers of the vastus lateralis are identified (**A**) and traced up to the vastus tubercle (**B**), looking immediately anterior to the lateral facet.

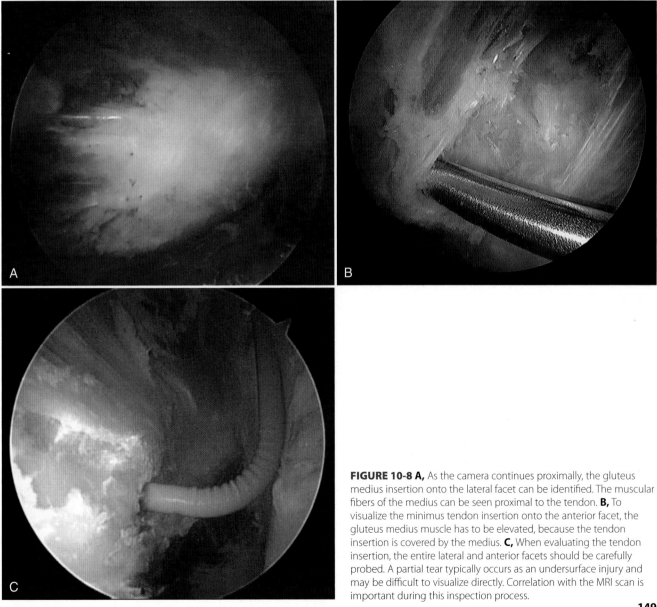

**FIGURE 10-8 A,** As the camera continues proximally, the gluteus medius insertion onto the lateral facet can be identified. The muscular fibers of the medius can be seen proximal to the tendon. **B,** To visualize the minimus tendon insertion onto the anterior facet, the gluteus medius muscle has to be elevated, because the tendon insertion is covered by the medius. **C,** When evaluating the tendon insertion, the entire lateral and anterior facets should be carefully probed. A partial tear typically occurs as an undersurface injury and may be difficult to visualize directly. Correlation with the MRI scan is important during this inspection process.

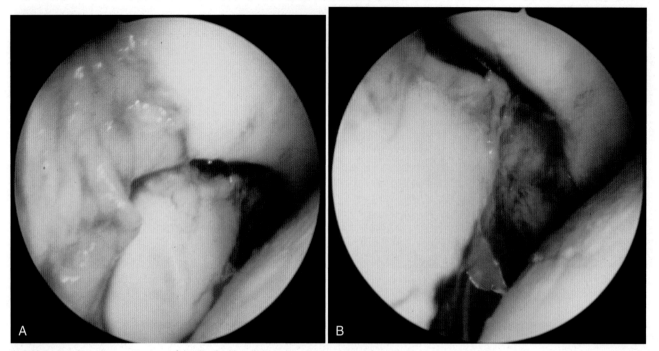

**FIGURE 10-9 A,** Arthroscopic view of the iliotibial band. **B,** Arthroscopic release of iliotibial band can be performed if necessary to decompress space or in the setting of symptomatic coxa saltans externus.

The technique for repairing a full-thickness tear of the abductor tendons is similar to that described for the rotator cuff. A thorough débridement of the trochanteric bursa is performed first to decompress the compartment and improve visualization (Fig. 10-10). The edges of the tear should be débrided, and clear margins around the tear should be demarcated (see Figs. 10-10C and D). Tears can be acute or chronic, and an assessment of reparability should be performed in an analogous fashion to that for rotator cuff tears by assessing the mobility of the torn edge and quality of the tissue (see Figs. 10-10E and F).

If the tear is repairable, the edges should be clearly identified and débrided to healthy viable tissue (Fig. 10-11A). Similarly, the anatomic footprint on the lateral facet should be cleared of soft tissue debris and decorticated to bleeding cancellous bone with a burr (see Figs. 10-11B and C). Suture anchors are then placed into the footprint using standard arthroscopic technique, typically through a small stab incision. A spinal needle or curved snap can be used to determine the ideal location and trajectory for anchor insertion, and confirmed with fluoroscopy (Fig. 10-12A). Placement of the anchor should be done under direct arthroscopic visualization (see Fig. 10-12B) and checked using fluoroscopy (see Fig. 10-12 C) to confirm an appropriate angle and location of insertion. Typically, two anchors will be sufficient to repair the anatomic footprint of a single tendon tear involving medius tears off the lateral facet. Adequate spacing of the anchors should allow for good bone stock between anchors (Fig. 10-13A and B).

Metallic anchors are frequently used because the bone quality of the trochanter is often good, and their position can be confirmed with fluoroscopy.

After anchors are placed, the sutures are passed sequentially through the free tendon edge using a suture-passing device (see Figs. 13C-F). Typically, the free edges of the tendon can be captured with a needle-penetrating device entering from the distal anterolateral accessory portal, and the suture can be placed in the midanterior portal. The second limb of the suture can be passed through the more distal fibers bordering on the edge of the vastus ridge using a standard suture-penetrating device. Careful suture management needs to be exercised to avoid suture entanglement. All suture passage and management should be performed through cannulas to avoid entrapment of overlying soft tissue.

Once the sutures have been passed and separated, sequential tying is performed using standard arthroscopic knot-tying technique (Fig. 10-14). Careful and complete evaluation of the tendon repair should be performed to confirm anatomic restoration of the tendon footprint and security of the repair.

Undersurface partial-thickness tears in the anterior medius tendon should be carefully assessed. If they are high-grade lesions, they may be converted into full-thickness tears with a full-radius shaver and repaired using the technique described earlier. Transtendon repairs may be performed in the setting of high-grade partial tears to avoid completion of the tear. Anchor placement and suture passage may be more difficult because visualization is impaired by the intact tendon.

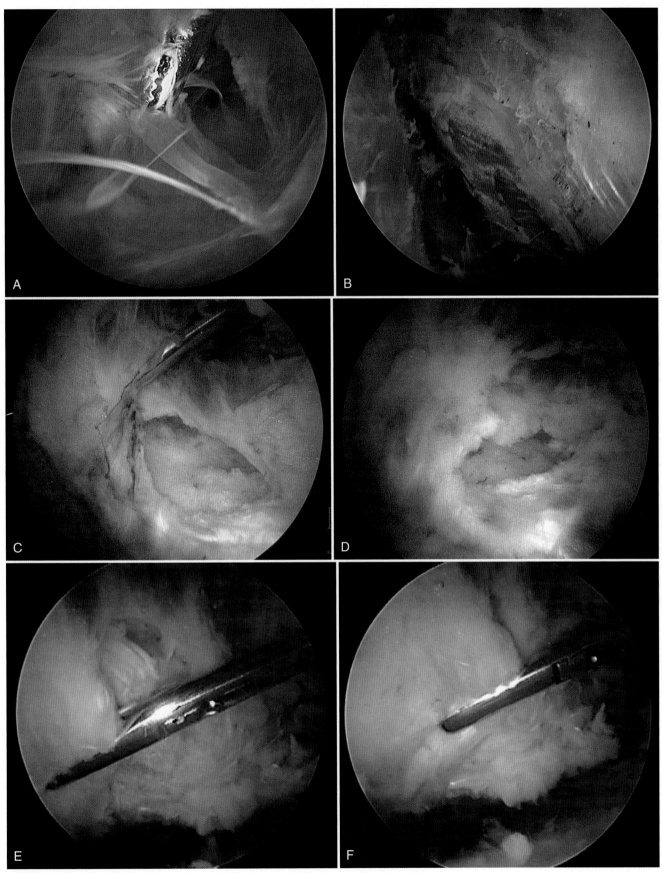

**FIGURE 10-10 A,** Thickened bursa is excised with the assistance of a motorized shaver to visualize and inspect the medius insertion fully. **B,** The gluteus medius muscle and tendon should be cleared of bursae. **C, D,** A full-thickness tear with retraction of the medius tendon is appreciated. **E, F,** The tear edges need to be demarcated clearly and the mobility of the tendon edge is tested.

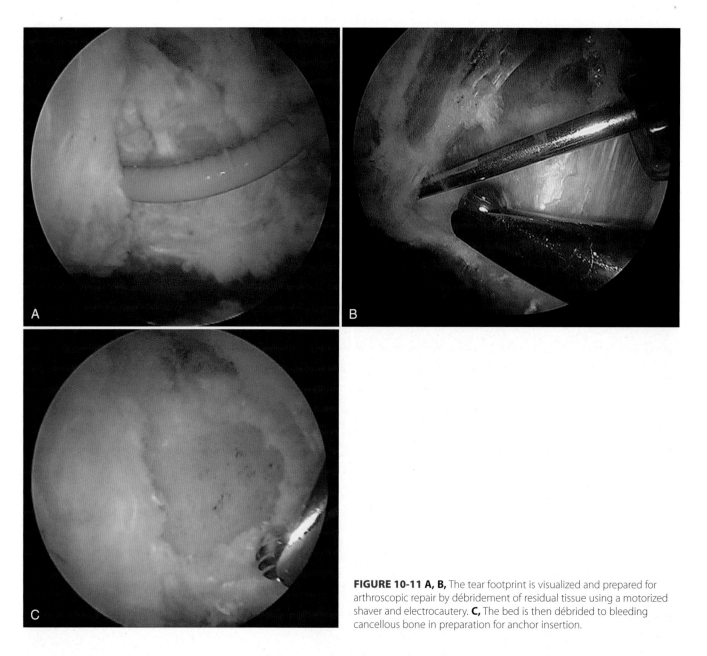

**FIGURE 10-11 A, B,** The tear footprint is visualized and prepared for arthroscopic repair by débridement of residual tissue using a motorized shaver and electrocautery. **C,** The bed is then débrided to bleeding cancellous bone in preparation for anchor insertion.

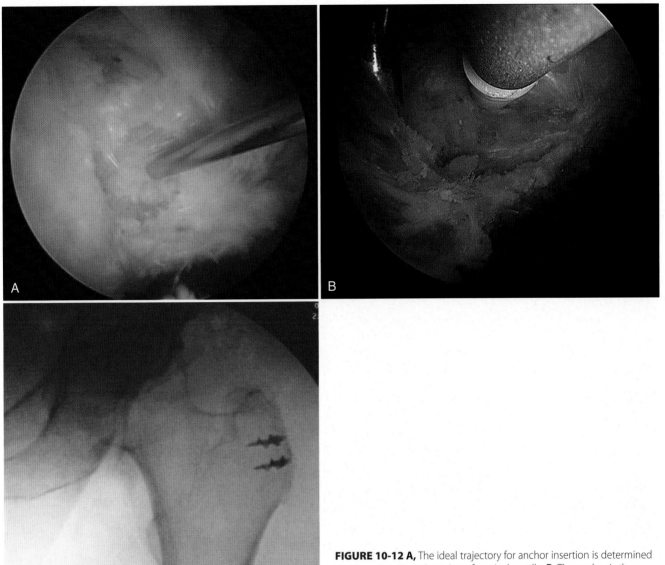

**FIGURE 10-12 A,** The ideal trajectory for anchor insertion is determined using percutaneous insertion of a spinal needle. **B,** The anchor is then placed through a small stab incision with this trajectory without difficulty. **C,** Anchor position along the facet can be confirmed with intraoperative fluoroscopy.

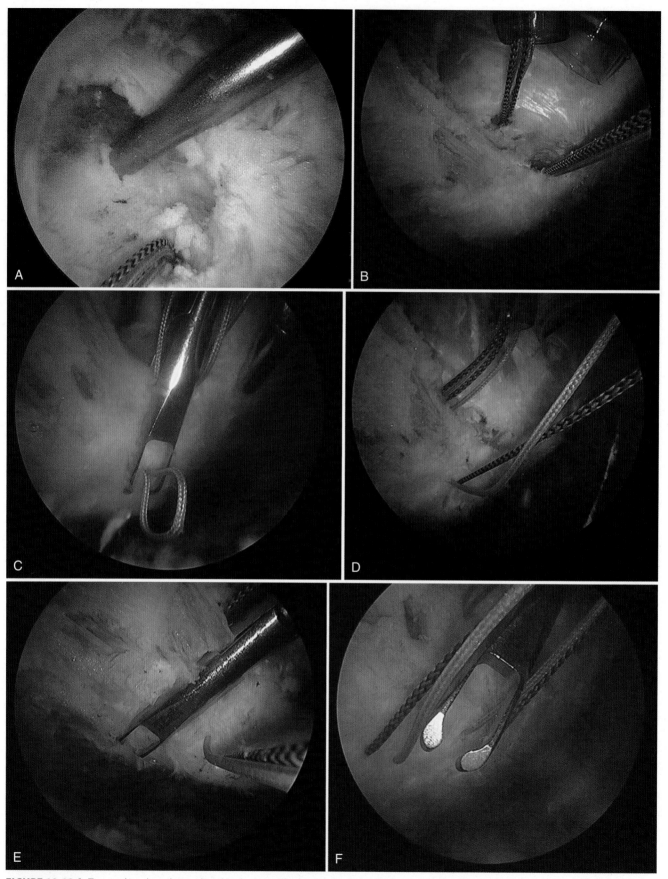

**FIGURE 10-13 A,** Two anchors have been placed in the lateral facet, each loaded with two sutures. **B,** Suture management is critical once the anchors are placed. All suture armanagement and tying should be performed through cannulas to avoid tissue incarceration within the suture. **C-G,** After the free edge of the tear is mobilized, a suture-passing device is used to grasp the retracted tendon edge. Simple or mattress sutures can be placed, depending on the tear configuration.

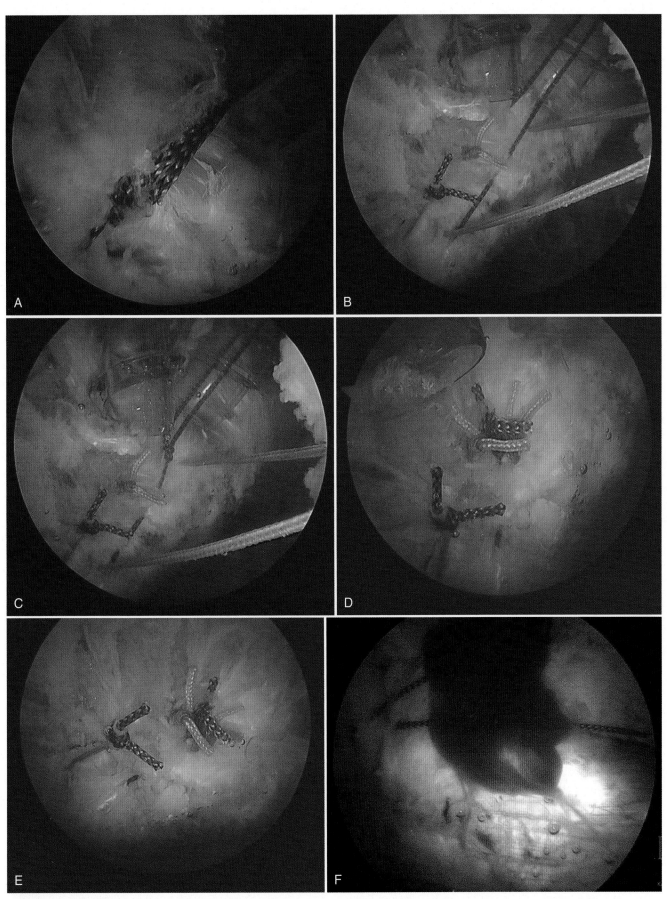

**FIGURE 10-14 A-F,** After sutures have been passed, arthroscopic knots are tied to repair the tendon to its footprint anatomically. Platelet-rich plasma can be delivered to the tendon-bone interface prior to knot tying for biologic augmentation of healing. The repair is probed to confirm excellent reduction and security.

## OUTCOMES

Voos and colleagues[20] have recently reviewed the short-term clinical outcomes of endoscopic gluteus medius tendon tear repairs performed by the senior author (BTK). Of 482 consecutive hip arthroscopies, 10 patients with medius tendon tears had endoscopic repair, with an average follow-up of 25 months. The patients' mean age was 50 years and all experienced persistent lateral hip discomfort and abductor weakness that was refractory to nonoperative measures. At final follow-up, all patients reported complete resolution of pain and had 5 of 5 abductor motor strength points on physical examination. Modified Harris hip scores at 1 year averaged 94 points and hip outcomes scores averaged 93 points.[20]

## POSTOPERATIVE REHABILITATION

The general goals of early postoperative rehabilitation are a normalized gait pattern with crutches and the abduction orthosis. The hip is placed in an abduction brace postoperatively to protect the hip from active abduction and passive adduction past neutral. No active abduction and internal rotation or passive adduction and external rotation are permitted for at least 6 weeks to protect the structural integrity of the repair. Passive hip flexion to 90 degrees and passive abduction, however, is permitted as tolerated. Weight bearing is restricted to 20 pounds of foot-flat on the involved extremity for the first 6 weeks postoperatively. Continuous passive motion is initiated immediately for 4 hours, as well as stationary biking for 20 minutes daily. This is continued for the first 4 to 6 weeks postoperatively to avoid adhesions. Scar massage of the portals is initiated after initial healing at 10 to 14 days postoperatively.

Isometric strengthening of hip extensors, adductors, and external rotators and quadriceps neuromuscular stimulation is initiated at 2 weeks postoperatively. Active hip strengthening is initiated at 4 to 6 weeks postoperatively, starting with isometric, submaximal hip flexion and quadriceps strengthening. Gradual progression to weight bearing as tolerated with crutches and progressive passive hip internal rotation, external rotation, and flexion to more than 90 degrees is allowed at 6 to 8 weeks postoperatively.

By 10 weeks, lower extremity strengthening, core strengthening, and proprioceptive training are progressed as tolerated. By 3 to 6 months, patients should be pain-free, with quadriceps and hamstring peak torque strength within 15% of the contralateral extremity on isokinetic testing. Furthermore, they should demonstrate a normal step-down test and score at least 85% or higher on the single-leg crossover triple hop for distance.

## REFERENCES

1. Bunker TD, Esler CN, Leach WJ. Rotator cuff tears of the hip. *J Bone Joint Surg Br.* 1997;79:618-620.
2. Kagan A 2nd. Rotator cuff tears of the hip. *Clin Orthop Relat Res.* 1999;(368):135-140.
3. Howell GE, Biggs RE, Bourne RB. Prevalence of abductor mechanism tears of the hips in patients with osteoarthritis. *J Arthroplasty.* 2001;16:121-123.
4. Bird PA, Oakley SP, Shnier R, Kirkham BW. Prospective evaluation of magnetic resonance imaging and physical examination findings in patients with greater trochanteric pain syndrome. *Arthritis Rheum.* 2001;44:2138-2145.
5. Beck M, Sledge JB, Gautier E, et al. The anatomy and function of the gluteus minimus muscle. *J Bone Joint Surg Br.* 2000;82:358-363.
6. Voos JE, Rudzki JR, Shindle MK et al. Arthroscopic anatomy and surgical techniques for peritrochanteric space disorders in the hip. *Arthroscopy.* 2007;23:1246.
7. Robertson WJ, Gardner MJ, Barker JU, et al. Anatomy and dimensions of the gluteus medius tendon insertion. *Arthroscopy.* 2008;24:130-136.
8. Dwek J, Pfirrman C, Stanley A, et al. MR imaging of the hip abductors: normal anatomy and commonly encountered pathology at the greater trochanter. *Magn Reson Imaging Clin North Am.* 2005;13:691-704.
9. Blankenbaker DG, Ullrick SR, Davis KW, et al. Correlation of MRI findings with clinical findings of trochanteric pain syndrome. *Skeletal Radiol.* 2008;37:903-909.
10. Cvitanic O, Henzie G, Skezas N, et al. MRI diagnosis of tears of the hip abductor tendons (gluteus medius and gluteus minimus). *AJR Am J Roentgenol.* 2004;182:137-143.
11. Lequesne M, Djian P, Vuillemin V, Mathieu P. Prospective study of refractory greater trochanter pain syndrome. MRI findings of gluteal tendon tears seen at surgery. Clinical and MRI results of tendon repair. *Joint Bone Spine.* 2008;75:458-464.
12. Craig RA, Jones DP, Oakley AP, Dunbar JD. Iliotibial band Z-lengthening for refractory trochanteric bursitis (greater trochanteric pain syndrome). *ANZ J Surg.* 2007;77:996-998.
13. Cormier G, Berthelot JM, Maugars Y; SRO (Société de Rhumatologie de l'Ouest). Gluteus tendon rupture is underrecognized by French orthopedic surgeons: results of a mail survey. *Joint Bone Spine.* 2006;73:411-413.
14. Ozçakar L, Erol O, Kaymak B, Aydemir N. An underdiagnosed hip pathology: apropos of two cases with gluteus medius tendon tears. *Clin Rheumatol.* 2004;23:464-466.
15. Connell DA, Bass C, Sykes CA, et al. Sonographic evaluation of gluteus medius and minimus tendinopathy. *Eur Radiol.* 2003;13:1339-1347.

16. Walsh G, Archibald CG. MRI in greater trochanter pain syndrome. *Australas Radiol*. 2003;47:85-87.

17. Lonner JH, Van Kleunen JP. Spontaneous rupture of the gluteus medius and minimus tendons. *Am J Orthop*. 2002 Oct;31: 579-581.

18. Kingzett-Taylor A, Tirman PF, Feller J, et al. Tendinosis and tears of gluteus medius and minimus muscles as a cause of hip pain: MR imaging findings. *AJR Am J Roentgenol*. 1999;173:1123-1126.

19. Chung CB, Robertson JE, Cho GJ, et al. Gluteus medius tendon tears and avulsive injuries in elderly women: imaging findings in six patients. *AJR Am J Roentgenol*. 1999;173:351-353.

20. Voos JE, Shindle MK, Pruett A, et al. Endoscopic repair of gluteus medius tendon tears of the hip. *Am J Sports Med*. 2009; 37:743-747.

# Computer-Assisted Surgery for Femoroacetabular Impingement

Asheesh Bedi ● Jérome Tonetti ● Laurence Chabanas ● Stéphane Lavallée ● Bryan T. Kelly

Femoroacetabular impingement (FAI) has recently been identified as the predominant cause of labral tears in the nondysplastic hip. Structural abnormalities in the morphology of the hip can limit motion and result in repetitive impact of the proximal femoral neck against the acetabular labrum and its adjacent cartilage. Bony impingement can result from a decrease in femoral head-neck offset (cam effect), an overgrowth of the bony acetabulum (pincer effect), excessive acetabular retroversion, or a combination of these deformities. Bony impingement with range of motion, particularly with internal rotation and flexion, can compromise the labrum and adjacent soft tissues, ultimately resulting in irreversible damage to the articular cartilage and early-onset joint degeneration. These recognized changes in the hip caused by impingement have all been associated with early-onset osteoarthritis of the young hip that was previously thought to be of idiopathic origin.

Arthroscopic treatment of FAI has grown in popularity during the last decade. Advantages include minimally invasive access to the hip joint, peripheral compartments, and associated soft tissues. Furthermore, arthroscopy allows for a dynamic intraoperative assessment and correction of the offending lesions. Although initially met with skepticism, the early results of arthroscopic treatment of FAI have shown favorable outcomes. A recent systematic review reported 67% to 100% good to excellent short-term clinical outcomes after arthroscopic treatment of hip impingement.[1] The long-term viability of these outcomes, however, is predicated on meticulous intraoperative evaluation and a thorough and accurate correction of impingement lesions on both the femoral and acetabular sides. Failure of arthroscopic techniques for FAI is most commonly associated with incomplete decompression of the associated bony anatomy.[2]

In this chapter, we first review the requirements for an ideal computer-assisted surgery (CAS) system dedicated to FAI by considering the major clinical issues that are encountered and also define our expectations for each of those issues. In the second section, we present an overview of the state-of-the-art systems and prototypes available, which indicate promising preliminary results that need to be further developed.

## REQUIREMENTS FOR A COMPUTER-ASSISTED SYSTEM

A computer-assisted surgery system dedicated to FAI could provide several advantages for the diagnosis and management of this disorder. Appropriate treatment of all sources of mechanical impingement, together with refixation of any viable labral tissue, is the recommended treatment intervention in symptomatic young adults to optimize the chances of a successful outcome and return to sport. The challenge remains, however, to diagnose, visualize, and eliminate the sources of impingement reliably, which can often be subtle and are only manifest with the use of provocative dynamic maneuvers.

### Preoperative Considerations

Cam impingement is the result of a loss of the normal sphericity of the femoral head from congenital, developmental, or post-traumatic changes in the shape of the proximal femur. The deformity typically occurs at the anterolateral aspect of the junction between the femoral head and neck, but can occur in any location around the circumference of the head-neck junction. Cam impingement results in a characteristic injury pattern to the transition zone cartilage of the acetabulum, where the labrum loses its structural attachment to the adjacent hyaline cartilage.

Pincer impingement results from overcoverage of the acetabulum, resulting in a specific pattern of labral degeneration as the overhanging bone on the acetabulum crushes the labrum during movement; this produces one or more cleavage planes of variable depth within the substance of the labrum. Subtypes of pincer morphology have been identified—focal anterosuperior overcoverage, coxa profunda, acetabular protrusio, and acetabular retroversion.[3] Identification of the specific type and location of pincer pathology is critical to developing an appropriate treatment plan that will reliably eliminate mechanical impingement postoperatively.

In addition to cam and pincer lesions, other geometric abnormalities can contribute to symptomatic hip pain and/or mechanical impingement. Recognizing these concomitant lesions is of tantamount importance to guide an appropriate surgical intervention. Femoral retroversion or excessive anteversion must be recognized. Coxa valga can also alter contact mechanics and kinematics of the hip. Acetabular dysplasia, including lateral and/or anterior undercoverage, is also not uncommon and can dramatically affect the load distribution and kinematics of the hip joint. It is essential to recognize the presence of these concomitant factors to develop an effective treatment plan for FAI.

In light of this geometric complexity, a CAS system could prove invaluable in the preoperative diagnostic and planning phases of FAI. The system could assimilate all the geometric considerations noted into a three-dimensional model. More importantly, however, such a system could subsequently subject the model to a dynamic mobility simulation to define any mechanical sources of impingement accurately. These simulations could be individualized based on patient activity level, ranging from simple gait to complex dance maneuvers or pivots required of competitive athletes. A virtual resection of varying degrees on both the femoral and acetabular sides could be performed and the dynamic analysis used to define the minimal resection on the femoral and acetabular sides that would be necessary to relieve mechanical impingement without adversely affecting the stability or kinematics of the joint. With these locations defined, this system could further indicate the ideal portals and trajectory to access these lesions while minimizing trauma to the periarticular soft tissues.

## Intraoperative Considerations

There are a number of technical issues associated with arthroscopic treatment of FAI that could substantially benefit from a computer assistance system. These include but are not limited to the following factors.

### Portals and Access

Currently, relatively universal portals are used to gain access into the intra-articular and peripheral compartments of the hip. Although these have been effective in treating cam and pincer lesions in the most typical locations, they can be less than optimal for more complex or large lesions. In particular, cam lesions that extend posteriorly and pincer lesions that extend far posteriorly or medially can be difficult to access safely with standard portals without placing neurovascular structures and the vascular supply to the femoral head at risk. Computer navigation systems could provide individualized novel portals to access these lesions safely and directly when necessary. Furthermore, trauma to the abductors and periarticular muscular envelope can be minimized by defining portals that use intermuscular planes and offer the shortest, most direct trajectory to the impingement lesions.

Another important consideration is exposure of the peripheral compartment. Current techniques use a moderate to large capsulotomy or capsulectomy to visualize the femoral neck adequately and define the margins of the cam lesion. This exposure is necessary with current techniques because successful treatment is predicated on thorough visualization and resection of the sources of impingement. However, such extensile exposure may not be without morbidity. Postoperative instability and hip dislocation have been reported after arthroscopic treatment of FAI. Furthermore, attempts at capsular closure after resection are technically very difficult and can be time-consuming, assuming sufficient tissue has been preserved. A computer assistance system may obviate the need and morbidity associated with such extensile exposures because the lesion can be precisely localized and resected through minimal capsular defects.

### Localization and Resection of Impingement Lesions

One of the most difficult aspects of the arthroscopic management of FAI remains localizing and defining the margins of the cam and pincer lesions. Even in the setting of an adequate exposure, the margins of the cam and pincer lesion are often not readily apparent. Experienced hip arthroscopists acknowledge that correlation of the location on preoperative imaging studies with intraoperative anatomy can be difficult, particularly with subtle and/or broad lesions that lack clearly discernible margins. Atypical cam lesions that extend posteriorly may not be immediately apparent and may require extensive internal rotation and accessory portals to perform an adequate resection.

Even if the locations of the cam and/or pincer lesions are accurately defined, the magnitude of resection that should be performed is perhaps even more difficult to define. Unfortunately, current techniques rely on the surgeon's judgment to define an adequate resection that will relieve mechanical impingement without compromising normal structural anatomy. Less experienced hip arthroscopists will tend to perform a less aggressive resection to avoid the risk of a femoral neck fracture or iatrogenic acetabular dysplasia from an overzealous resection. Unfortunately, this tendency leads to a high risk for residual impingement and unfavorable long-term outcomes. On the other hand, aggressive resections that extend beyond the margins of the cam lesion can compromise the cortical support of the native femoral neck and precipitate femoral neck fracture, a significant and potentially devastating postoperative complication. In addition, errant overresection of a pincer lesion on the acetabular side can result in iatrogenic undercoverage and dysplasia.

A computer assistance system could address both these technical issues reliably in the hands of adept and inexperienced hip arthroscopists. The system could merge preoperative imaging findings with real-time intraoperative anatomy, helping the surgeon to define the margins of the lesions unequivocally. Furthermore, the system could provide feedback to guide a complete resection to the appropriate depth while avoiding risk to native structures that do not contribute to the mechanical impingement. Such a system would decrease the dependence of intraoperative surgical judgment to define an adequate and precise resection of all pathology arbitrarily, and allow favorable outcomes to be reliably achieved, even by relatively inexperienced surgeons.

### Fluoroscopy

Current techniques in hip arthroscopy rely extensively on intraoperative fluoroscopy throughout the procedure. It is used to guide portal placement and access into the intra-articular compartment, and is also a "poor man's" guide to localize cam and pincer lesions and confirm adequate resection. Unfortunately, this modality is certainly operator-dependent and limited by the quality of the images that can be obtained intraoperatively, given the limitations of patient positioning. Furthermore, under the best of circumstances, fluoroscopy provides two-dimensional feedback for three-dimensional pathology and can provide limited information regarding the adequacy of resection in multiple planes. In addition, the extensive use of fluoroscopy intraoperatively certainly exposes the patient and surgeon to radiation that can be substantial over the course of a surgical career.

A computer assistance system may significantly reduce the need for intraoperative fluoroscopy and reduce the risks associated with its use. The feedback provided by the system could guide safe and direct portal placement and allow the surgeon to perform an adequate and thorough resection of the cam and/or pincer lesions based on more accurate, three-dimensional data that are obtained preoperatively.

### Dynamic Assessment

Perhaps one of the greatest advantages of a computer assistance system is its ability to provide immediate feedback regarding the precise and accurate treatment of FAI via dynamic simulation. FAI is a dynamic pathology that manifests itself symptomatically during provocative maneuvers of the hip that are unique to individual patient activities. Current arthroscopic techniques do not allow for a complete dynamic evaluation of the recontoured hip because of constraints of patient positioning, instrumentation, and swelling caused by fluid extravasation during the procedure. A computer assistance system could assess the kinematics of the hip intraoperatively to confirm that the performed resection has eliminated mechanical impingement with previously symptomatic maneuvers.

## STATE OF THE ART OF COMPUTER-ASSISTED SURGERY

### Methods

Many CAS technologies have been developed over the last 20 years, with applications in orthopedic surgery since the early 1990s.[4-6] First, CAS systems depend on the type of patient information that is used. Most systems for total knee and hip surgery use image-free technology in which an optical or magnetic localization system is used to collect bony anatomic reference points intraoperatively. No computed tomography (CT) or magnetic resonance imaging (MRI) scanning is necessary. An extension of those methods considers the use of deformable statistical models to fit the patient anatomy from a collection of surface points.[7] In the domain of FAI, none of those image-free techniques have yet given satisfactory results. Because of the complex pathology, preoperative three-dimensional images seem to be necessary. Both CT and MRI have pros and cons, but technically the use of preoperative CT scans provides reliable and accurate contours of bones that make possible automatic processing. So far, extraction of bone and cartilage surfaces from MRI scans can be only achieved manually with semiautomated tools. In the ideal world, fused CT and MRI scans in three dimensions would be the best option, CT because it is accurate and reliable and can be processed automatically, and MRI because it visualizes soft tissues and can be registered automatically to CT images. In practice, CT seems to be a sufficient means to address the requirements indicated at reasonable cost but the debate remains open.

Second, at the planning stage, a CAS system requires a clear definition of an objective to be reached. For instance, a bone cut at 90 degrees of the tibial mechanical axis is a standard target in computer-assisted total knee surgery. For FAI, the target is much more complex and much research needs to be accomplished before a precise definition of the best planning criteria can be determined automatically. However, a computer can be used interactively to predict the impingement area for simulated resections on images and the corresponding range of motion of the hip. Individual simulation can be achieved for each patient to understand the complexity of the pathology, take into account femoral neck retroversion, select the relative area of resection on both femur and acetabulum that need correction, simulate portals to reach the selected area, and obtain a true rehearsal of surgery prior to any incision more globally.

Third, a registration method must be used to match the preoperative images and planning with the intraoperative position of the femur and acetabulum during surgery.[8] A mandatory step of any navigation system is to attach trackers to the bones; this is usually accomplished by inserting one 6- or two 3-mm pins in the greater trochanter for the femur and iliac crest for the pelvis. With most ergonomic systems, this takes only a few seconds and has no associated significant risk. These reference trackers can be placed anywhere but must not move during surgery. At that stage, the registration process can start. There are several known methods, including the following:

- Digitization of bone surface landmarks or surface areas using a calibrated probe equipped with a tracker.

    These landmarks can be directly paired to points identified in preoperative three-dimensional data, or a distance minimization algorithm can be applied to compute the matching transform. This method is usually fast and does not require any other processing from the acquired data. The issue in our case is to digitize bony landmarks percutaneously, which requires a dedicated needle.

- Fluoroscopy can be used to acquire intraoperative images and match them with the preoperative data set.

    This requires the installation of a calibration device on the C-arm and some x-ray images to achieve the registration. This technique is usually accurate but may fail when the quality of fluoroscopic images is poor.

- Ultrasound is a noninvasive modality that enables access to difficult areas.

    The ultrasound probe is equipped with a tracker to localize the surface segmented in the images and match it to the preoperative data. It is the most elegant and fast solution for registration.[9] We have obtained promising results in that area but industrial development of a system that can be used in clinical practice has not been accomplished so far.

- Intraoperative three-dimensional fluoroscopic imaging is a recent technique that can be used to register the CT or MRI scan based on planning in a stable, precise, and robust manner.

    In addition, this provides postoperative control with three-dimensional images. However, it is not yet available in most operating rooms.

- The final stage is the intraoperative navigation, which can be done once the registration process has succeeded.

    Surgical instruments, such as reamers or shavers, can be equipped with trackers. Usually, the tip and the axis of the instrument are calibrated and its current position is displayed in the preoperative image volume in real time. In conventional navigation systems, the tip of the instrument is displayed as a cross hair on three orthogonal reconstructed CT images passing through the tip of the instrument. In the case of FAI, such display is not sufficient. The navigation must take more dedicated formats, including a display of the tip with respect to the anatomy labeled with clock sectors. In addition, the target area to be resected needs to be delineated during the planning phase.

Several research groups have started to develop and evaluate computer-assisted technologies to address specific issues of FAI surgery. The different teams and their work, discussed in the following sections, range from diagnosis to planning and modeling, and finally intraoperative navigation. This re-

view does not pretend to be exhaustive but will present some of the state-of-the-art research currently being undertaken.

## Preoperative Assistance

A group at the Müller Institute in Bern, Switzerland, has developed a platform to analyze the hip joint in three dimensions, using two-dimensional x-rays of the pelvis.[10] A combination of anteroposterior (AP) and lateral radiographs are integrated into a projection model to create a virtual three-dimensional reconstruction of the pelvis. The goal of this computation is to standardize the measured radiographic parameters, especially the caudocranial femoral head coverage used in the diagnosis of impingement. The main contribution of this work is a standardization of the pelvis orientation that was developed to take into account individual tilt and rotation variability. This absolute reference is computed from a correction of the radiographic orientation based on anatomic and radiographic parameters describing the morphology of the hip. A dedicated software (Hip²Norm) has been developed for that purpose. A validation study was conducted to evaluate the results statistically and quantitatively on 60 cadavers and qualitatively on 51 patients. Depending on the measured parameters, the interpretation of the results showed a satisfactory analysis. Except for the restriction of being applicable only to spherical joint configurations, the method was proved accurate and valuable to help in the diagnosis of the acetabular morphology from two-dimensional radiographs.

Several computer-assisted systems have been developed to implement a kinematic modeling of the hip joint to plan the surgery and simulate the postoperative situation. These planning systems are based on preoperative imaging, using CT or MRI.

A group from Geneva University has addressed this preoperative planning issue with a four-stage method.[11] The method developed by this group was intended to help the surgeon in diagnosis, localization of the impingement area, and determination of the area and amount of bone to be resected to regain a satisfactory range of motion. The first stage is the reconstruction of a three-dimensional surface model of the joint, femur, and acetabulum. MRI was used and different slice thicknesses were considered, according to the requested accuracy at different levels of the joint. Manual segmentation of bony contours was performed and three-dimensional surface models were reconstructed. The second stage is the integration of joint kinematics in the surface model to simulate circumduction motion. The main issue with this step is the correct determination of the hip center of rotation, which is done with an iterative procedure. The simulation of the bone reshaping is the third stage of the planning and involves three procedures.

The femoral head is first reshaped by fitting a sphere on its three-dimensional surface, which defines the areas out of the sphere as the impingement zone to be resected. An impingement test simulation is performed to determine the acetabular rim that produces overcoverage of the femoral head. The simulation of the acetabular resection is done manually by intersecting the three-dimensional surface model with planes until the impingement has been reduced. Periacetabular osteotomy lines can also be simulated manually by fitting a controlled curve over the surface of the model. The last step is the computation of the range of motion (ROM). Several joint motions including flexion and extension, rotation, and abduction and adduction can be combined and impingement detection tools can predict the postoperative range of motion after virtual surgery. The developed system is based only on the MRI data from a group of healthy volunteers. It provides the main hip kinematic factors defining the ROM. However, the team that implemented this program does not claim any cadaveric validation or clinical trials.

Another important work on planning and simulation of the treatment has been done by another group from Bern, Switzerland.[12] The aim of this system is to provide a tool to help the surgeon better assess the preoperative situation of the hip joint and to plan the most appropriate correction to solve the patient's femoroacetabular impingement. The software developed, HipMotion, is based on a patient's preoperative CT scans, enabling a real three-dimensional analysis of the joint. As in the work discussed earlier,[11] the patient's three-dimensional model is reconstructed from preoperative three-dimensional image data. A collision detection algorithm is applied during simulated joint motion to determine the regions of impingement. A quantification of the trimming of bony structures is displayed and can be adjusted. The simulation of postoperative ROM is then computed after these virtual resections have been applied. The automatic computation of the range of motion from a reconstructed three-dimensional joint model has been validated on sawbones and cadaveric hips by comparing the simulations given by the preoperative analysis HipMotion software with actual measurements obtained using a commercially available navigation system from BrainLAB (Feldkirchen, Germany). Reproducibility and reliability were assessed from the results, except for external rotation measurements that showed a moderate similarity. The software had then been used for a pilot clinical study, in which the ROM of a control group was compared with FAI patients. From that quantitative study, it could be shown that the ROM measurements did correspond to what was described more qualitatively in the literature. A significant difference in flexion, abduction, internal rotation, and internal rotation at 90 degrees of flexion angle was detected between the control and study groups, with these angles being significantly reduced for the impingement patients. It could also be shown that the impingement zones automatically computed from the software precisely matched the reported anterosuperior labral and chondral lesion areas observed intraoperatively.

The goal of such preoperative planning systems is to analyze the preoperative impingement situation accurately and plan the location and amount of bony resection, therefore save time in the operating room, by knowing how to address the problem better. However, none of this research discussed has been combined with an effective intraoperative navigation system. The next stage of such programs would be the actual implementation of the planned resections during surgery.

## Intraoperative Navigation

The next step in computer-assisted FAI surgery is intraoperative tracking and control of the resection(s). Arthroscopy can benefit valuably from navigation systems, which could then address issues of over- or undercorrection. CT-based navigation systems have been used clinically to evaluate the potential improvements brought by intraoperative assistance to arthroscopic FAI procedures. The most challenging issues of such systems is the registration of preoperative images of the patient to the intraoperative situation. Both research studies discussed next used an adapted, commercially available system based on fluoro-CT registration to navigate hip impingement.

One group, based in Boston, published preliminary results using this system for combined impingement types.[13] The system was used for acetabular rim and femoral head-neck offset correction. Four patients were reported to have undergone this computer-assisted procedure combined with conventional arthroscopy. The intraoperative registration was successful for all cases and actual tracking of the surgical instruments was performed. However, this system does not allow for intraoperative quantification of bone resection during the procedure, nor can the ROM gain from the current débridement be assessed.

More recently, a similar system was used for a prospective clinical study by a group in Wolhusen, Switzerland.[14] The purpose of that study was the evaluation of the impact of a CT-based navigation system from BrainLab on the accuracy of the head-neck offset correction for patients undergoing an arthroscopic procedure for a cam-type impingement lesion. It also sought to evaluate the impact of offset restoration accuracy on early clinical outcomes. The clinical team used preoperative and postoperative MRI scans to evaluate the correction of the alpha angle. A postoperative angle of less than 50 degrees or a correction of more than 20 degrees was considered a successful correction. The intraoperative navigation system also required a preoperative CT scan. The registration was again performed through fluoroscopic image matching. The tracking of surgical instruments by the navigation system was displayed as different three-dimensional views and two-dimensional slices of the patient's femoral head model. The distance of the instrument tip to the bone surface was computed and displayed, allowing an approximate quantification of the actual bone resection depth. The analysis of the study cases showed no significant statistical difference in the successful correction rate in the navigated or non-navigated groups. Both groups showed 24% insufficient correction of the offset. An average of 25 minutes of extra operating time was observed for the navigated procedures. The current state of the presented CT fluoroscopy–based navigation system does not show any improvement in the correction rate. Moreover, the display of the tracking stage and the presented measures do not help the surgeon assess the amount of bony resection better. Finally, because no preoperative planning can be integrated into the system, there is no predefined target to be reached. The main inconvenience of this adapted system is that it is not fully dedicated to the assistance of FAI arthroscopic procedures. Hence, it cannot provide the specific features required to observe the expected improvements from a navigation system.

Finally, another solution based on computer-assisted encoder linkage navigation concept has been proposed by a team at Carnegie Mellon University (Pittsburgh).[15] That system claims to provide assistance first during portal placement to avoid neurovascular structures and then tracking of the surgical instruments. The advantages of using an encoder linkage structure for intraoperative navigation are the elimination of occlusion and distortion problems commonly known with optical and electromagnetic systems. Patients' preoperative three-dimensional image data have to be obtained from CT or MRI scans or model reconstruction from x-rays. A stiff base pin used to support and attach the tracking linkage is fixed to the patient's bone and triangulation from intraoperative x-rays is used to register preoperative data to the patient. The linkage arm is mounted to the base pin on one extremity, and the arthroscope or surgical instrument is attached to the other extremity. Two linkage chains are required if tracking of both the arthroscope and surgical tool is to be done. The visualization software displays the relative position of the instrument tip and axis relative to the patient structures. When the arthroscope is navigated, a simulated arthroscopic view is computed that can then be compared with the actual arthroscopic image. A mechanical bench setting has been designed to test the linkage device positioning accuracy. The positioning error has two sources, intrinsic encoder resolution and initialization method of the chain. The overall chain accuracy was show to be within an average of about 5 mm, mainly because of initialization process sensitivity, which needs to be further improved. It was reported that this system provided valuable information while offering a good flexibility required by the narrow space of arthroscopic surgery. All experiences are based only on a phantom hip joint.

## Discussion of Current Research Studies

Although promising results have been obtained, none of the research programs described here has yet been offered in a commercial version dedicated to FAI. The demand from experienced and nonexperienced surgeons is very high and the needs are clearly expressed. There are a number of reasons for this disappointing situation.

First, the industry is more focused on CAS techniques for large implants because of the market size. The domain of FAI is still in its infancy and long-term proven clinical results have not yet been published, which represent high risks for the industry. In addition, the existing technologies of navigation are not mature enough to address the current challenges without adding complexity and losing time; this is a very critical point, because most existing navigation systems are too cumbersome, time-consuming, expensive, and non–user-friendly, although each manufacturer claims the opposite.

Finally, modeling our clinical problems into a technical system is not trivial, and many issues remain. These dictate extensive work for precise definition of requirements; hopefully we made this clear in the first section of this chapter. Therefore, there is an urgent need to provide a dedicated solution that meets all defined requirements. In that respect, our group is working to develop a new generation of CAS solutions that integrates planning and navigation functions, with the major goals of being user-friendly and not adding operative time. Figures 11-1 and 11-2 illustrate this new concept under development by A[2] Surgical (La Tronche, France).

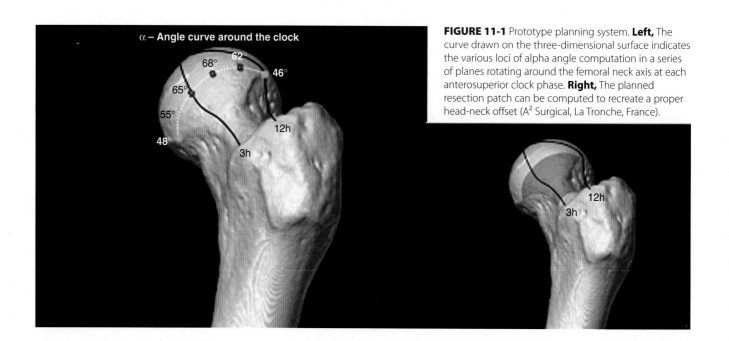

**FIGURE 11-1** Prototype planning system. **Left,** The curve drawn on the three-dimensional surface indicates the various loci of alpha angle computation in a series of planes rotating around the femoral neck axis at each anterosuperior clock phase. **Right,** The planned resection patch can be computed to recreate a proper head-neck offset (A[2] Surgical, La Tronche, France).

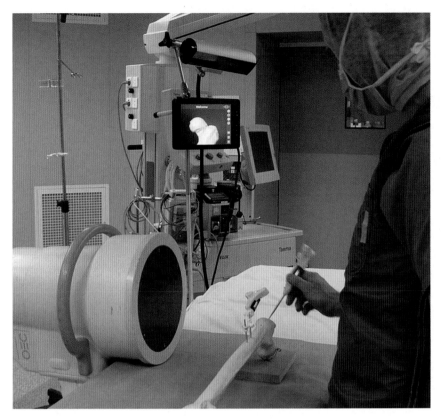

**FIGURE 11-2** Prototype navigation system. This miniature navigation station is attached to the surgical table and locates in real time the position of the burr in correlation with the target surface areas as defined during the planning phase

## CONCLUSIONS

With our increasing understanding of the mechanical sources of prearthritic hip pain, the complexities surrounding the diagnosis of FAI has become apparent. No longer is it as simple as stating that there is a cam lesion, a pincer lesion, or a combination of both. Rather, a multitude of underlying anatomic considerations all contribute equally to the dynamic and the static loads to which cartilage surfaces are subjected. Computer navigation will greatly improve our ability not only to make impingement diagnoses with greater precision, but also to correct impingement pathology more accurately.

Complete analysis of the bony anatomy includes circumferential measurements of femoral head-neck offset, acetabular relationships between the anterior and posterior walls, analysis of acetabular coverage in the sagittal and coronal planes, and rotational (version) and angular (varus-valgus) measurements of the femoral neck on the shaft. Each of these parameters will have an effect on the mechanical load across the hip joint, and each must be factored into the surgical solution for the impinging hip. It is naïve to believe that these complexities can be resolved with visual estimation alone. A global and complete approach can be accomplished only with the assistance of computer navigation. Our ability to improve the accuracy and precision of the diagnosis and treatment of FAI will be reflected in continued improvement in patient outcomes and increased longevity of the native hip.

## REFERENCES

1. Bedi A, Chen N, Robertson W, Kelly BT. The management of labral tears and femoroacetabular impingement of the hip in the young, active patient. *Arthroscopy.* 2008;24:1135-1145.
2. Heyworth BE, Shindle MK, Voos JE, et al. Radiologic and intraoperative findings in revision hip arthroscopy. *Arthroscopy.* 2007;23:1295-1302.
3. Beck M, Kalhor M, Leunig M, Ganz R. Hip morphology influences the pattern of damage to the acetabular cartilage: femoroacetabular impingement as a cause of early osteoarthritis of the hip. *J Bone Joint Surg Br.* 2005;87:1012-1018.
4. Lavallee S, Bainville E, Bricault I. An overview of computer-integrated surgery and therapy (CIST). In: Udupa J, Herman J, eds. 3D Imaging In Medicine, 2nd ed. Boca Raton, Fla: CRC Press; 2000:207-264.
5. Tonetti J, Carrat L, Lavallée S, et al. Percutaneous iliosacral screw placement using image guided techniques. *Clin Orthop Rel Res.* 1998;(354):103-110.
6. Dessenne V, Lavallée S, Orti R, et al. Computer-assisted knee anterior cruciate ligament reconstruction: first clinical tests. *J Im Guided Surg.* 1995;1:59-64.
7. Stindel E, Briard JL, Merloz P, et al. Bone morphing: 3D morphological data for total knee arthroplasty. *Comput Aided Surg.* 2002;7:156-168.
8. Lavallée S. Registration for computer integrated surgery: methodology, state of the art. In: Taylor R, Lavallee S, Burdea G, Mosges R, eds. Computer Integrated Surgery. Cambridge, Mass: MIT Press: 1996:77-97.
9. Kilian P, Plaskos C, Parratte S, et al. New visualization tools: computer vision and ultrasound for MIS navigation. *Int J Med Robot Comput Assist Surg.* 2008;4:23-31.

10. Tannast M, Mistry S, Steppacher SD, et al. Radiographic analysis of femoroacetabular impingement with hip. 2. Norm-reliable and validated. *J Orthop Res.* 2008;26:1199-1205.

11. Kang MJ, Sadri H, Magnenat-Thalmann N. Computer-assisted pre-operative planning for hip joint-preserving surgery. Paper presented at: 5th Annual Meeting of the International Society for Computer Assisted Orthopaedic Surgery; June 2005; Helsinki, Finland.

12. Tannast M, Kubiak-Langer M, et al. Noninvasive three-dimensional assessment of femoroacetabular impingement. *J Orthop Res.* 2007;25:122-131.

13. Murphy SB, Ecker TM, Tuma G, Haimerl M. Arthroscopic percutaneous computer assisted FAI relief using a new method of CT-fluoro registration. Paper presented at: 7th Annual Meeting of the International Society for Computer Assisted Orthopaedic Surgery; June 2007; Heidelberg, Germany.

14. Brunner A, Horisberger M, Herzog R. Evaluation of a computer tomography-based navigation system prototype for hip arthroscopy in the treatment of femoroacetabular cam impingement. *Arthroscopy.* 2009;25:382-391.

15. Monahan E, Shimada K. Computer-aided navigation for arthroscopic hip surgery using encoder linkages for position tracking. *Int J Med Robotics Comput Assist Surg.* 2006;2:271-278.

# Index

Note: Page numbers followed by f refer to figures; page numbers followed by t refer to tables; pages numbers followed by b refer to boxes.